Ayurveda

The Science of Life

By

Dr. Alda Sainfort

Acknowledgement

The author of this book acknowledges her supporter and those who contributed positively to the writing of this book. she would like to express her most sincere and deepest gratitude to her husband, Emmanuel Sainfort; her three children: Maggie Garcia, Majnheiv Sainfort, and Majnisharah Sainfort; her Granddaughter Neomi Alda Garcia; her father, Walvidace Hilaire, relatives, family, and friends; and lasty to Dr. Aparna Bapat, president of the Ayurvedic Association of Florida (AAF) who has been a wonderful supporter, instructor and mentor.

"My experience at Advanced Healing Wellness Center has been life-changing in the most beautiful and positive way. The variety of services offered with the utmost attention and care has given my family and me true holsistic healing. My healing has taken place on many levels, improving my entire well-being. I highly recommend Advanced Healing Wellness Center in Pembroke Pines for all your health and wellness needs, physical, emotional, mental, nutritional, and spiritual."

Jade

Table of Contents

Chapter 1

Introduction to Ayurveda

What is Ayurveda?

Ayurveda—the mother of all healing sciences—is the world's oldest medicinal system that emerged in India about 5,000 years ago. It is perhaps the longest-surviving tradition in the history of humankind, which has been practiced continually and is still popular today.

Ayurveda comes from two Sanskrit words: Ayur (life) and Veda (knowledge or science). It loosely translates as the knowledge of life or the science of life. Originally evolved as a form of personalized medical care, the primary goal of Ayurveda is not to fight diseases. It is a full and comprehensive approach to better health that seeks to enhance wellness through greater self-awareness and a preventive lifestyle.

The Ayurvedic way of life seeks to create balance in the body and mind, with the ultimate goal of bringing self-actualization—a heightened state of awareness that enables an individual to live life at its fullest and realize one's full potential.

Origin of Ayurveda: A long history of healing

Ayurvedic wisdom recorded in classic texts results from thousands of years of scientific observation, exploration, reasoning, debate, and trial and error. The origin of Ayurveda can be traced back to the oral traditions of ancient India when learned sages, who also served as healers, started observing how the mind and body can self-heal if the natural balance is restored.

They started observing how everything in the universe is connected. Scholars started asking and debating questions like why one health issue often leads to another, how food impacts the way we feel and act, why certain activities are more suitable at specific times of the day, how seasons affect our health, why medicines do not work equally for everyone, and what makes us unique.

The vast repository of knowledge gathered in this way passed through generations of healers, many of whom added their own observation to the practice, at times questioning, refining, and modifying previously established theories.

Over time, Ayurveda became a comprehensive lifestyle and self-care practice, encompassing almost every aspect of living. Nutrition, yoga, meditation, aromatherapy, daily routine, seasonal routine, stress management techniques, use of medicinal herbs and spices, and healthy cooking and eating practices—all became a part of the practice and were collectively known as the Ayurvedic way of life.

Ayurvedic learning continued to spread through oral traditions for centuries before it was finally documented in the fourth book of Vedas—the Atharva Veda—a voluminous collection documenting several diseases with their treatments.

The period from the second to the sixth century witnessed remarkable developments in science and medicine. Some major works, including the *Charaka Samhita*, the *Sushruta Samhita*, and the *Ashtanga Hridayam*, were produced around this period, enriching, and expanding the scope of ayurvedic medicine.

Centuries of refinement have imparted this ancient way of life a rational and logical basis, which has stood the test of time. Even now, scientists worldwide are actively exploring the principles of Ayurvedic medicine, which may provide an alternative way to look at health and help address the mounting challenges of modern times. Recent investigations have validated the preventive efficacy of ayurvedic herbs and self-care practices, especially the ones related to mental health and lifestyle diseases.

Philosophy and principles of Ayurveda

The core principle of Ayurveda is that prevention is always better than curative measures. Not just prevention, it proposes a way of living that seeks to consciously promote health through personalized self-care practices, such as mindful eating, adequate sleep, daily routine, discipline, seasonal regimen, periodic detox, yoga, meditation, and adaptogen herbs.

Health is a broad concept referring to optimal physical, mental, emotional, social, and spiritual well-being that enables an individual to feel her best. Ayurveda encourages us to live a balanced life that minimizes stress in all forms and brings contentment.

Although it is a holistic system of medicine, therapeutic interventions are considered secondary in Ayurveda. The focus is on cultivating a habit of mindful living that helps build immunity, vitality, mental calm, and emotional resilience.

How Ayurveda fits into modern life

The beauty of Ayurveda is that despite being subject to constant change throughout history, the core philosophy of this ancient practice still holds today. Its timeless principle emphasizing prevention and health promotion is more significant now than ever.

At a time when the world is trying to recover from a pandemic, anxiety and depression are more common than ever, obesity and nutritional deficiency exist side by side, and indiscriminate use of drugs has led to drug resistance. We are losing real connections in an increasingly virtual world; Ayurveda can show us how to reclaim our health and improve self-connection.

Yoga is the sister science of Ayurveda

Ayurveda and yoga originated around the same time and are rooted in the Vedas, one of the earliest pieces of world literature dealing with health, philosophy, medicine, and spirituality. But the connection between these sister sciences is not only historical; they also have a shared goal and belief system. They complement each other in every way and are best practiced together.

Both Ayurveda and yoga believe that every human being (microcosm) is a small part or reflection of the universe (macrocosm) that represents the bigger picture. We are made up of the same elements and are moved by the same energies that govern everything around us. Only by living in harmony with nature can we achieve perfect health, balance, and peace of mind.

4

But while yoga is philosophical and spiritual in its approach, Ayurveda is a full-fledged system of medicine that integrates various components of yoga into its practice.

A comprehensive system of medicine: How Ayurvedic healing works

Ayurveda complements modern medicine

Modern medicine is undeniably one of the greatest achievements of humankind, which has secured a better quality of life for many. But it has not been able to address the growing burden of lifestyle diseases and mental health issues. Embracing an Ayurvedic way of life can help bridge this gap and offer a holistic solution to these problems.

Ayurveda's health-promoting practices, like proper diet, routine, exercise, and stress management techniques, can improve healing and sustain the benefits of medicines. Moreover, its focus on immunity and self-care can also reduce the dependence on medications, which may come with numerous side effects and contribute to drug resistance.

Ayurvedic medicine is highly personalized

Conventional medicine follows a one-size-fits-all approach that is unfortunately not very helpful. It assumes there is one medicine, one treatment plan, and one form of therapy that will work for everyone. This belief arises from a notion that views a person as a body of flesh, blood, and bones.

On the other hand, Ayurveda views a person as a total of four parts: body, mind, soul, and senses. It recognizes that every person is unique and needs personalized care. There is a saying in Ayurveda that "nothing is right for everyone; everything is right for someone."

When diagnosed with a condition, your Ayurvedic doctor considers two things before outlining a treatment plan: your original constitution (Prakriti) and current dosha imbalance (Vikriti). So, even if two persons suffer from the same disease, their treatment plans may differ.

More than medicines

Healing in Ayurveda is not all about treating the symptoms. In this ancient healing science, diseases are viewed as imbalances. Every health problem is a sign of an underlying imbalance, and treating the symptoms may not help unless the balance is restored.

Ayurveda believes that treating only the symptoms will leave the person vulnerable to other related health problems in the near future. It tries to identify and address the root cause that had started and facilitated the disease in the first place.

Once the cause is identified, a personalized treatment plan is outlined. Along with medicines, the prescription includes diet and lifestyle modifications that help accelerate healing and prevent future health complications.

Ayurvedic therapies typically include:

- Dietary changes
- Cleansing and purification programs
- Rejuvenating therapy with medicated oils
- Restorative yoga poses
- Meditation and breathing exercises
- Aromatherapy with essential oils

- Immune-boosting herbs and decoctions
- Calming Herbal teas
- Therapies for aiding the nervous system

Ayurvedic medicines are not home remedies. In fact, it is treated on par with medical sciences in its home country India. Indian Ayurvedic doctors undergo institutionalized medical training, which is a state-recognized bachelor's degree program of five and a half years duration.

It is also important to note that Ayurvedic medicines and therapies are not always safe, although they come from natural sources. They also have side effects, especially if taken in improper ways. Just like other forms of medicine, Ayurvedic remedies should also be taken (or performed) under the supervision of experts.

CHAPTER 2

Fundamental Elements of Nature

Panchamahabhutas: The five great elements

The theory of Panchamahabhutas, meaning the five great elements, is a foundational concept in Ayurveda. Ayurvedic perception of the universe (macrocosm), matter (microcosm), life and its diverse forms (interaction of both), and forces that govern them all—everything begins with five elements.

Elements also provide the basis for studying the human body and mind—and how we interact with the larger world surrounding us. The nature of this interaction is believed to influence health and disease directly, and this understanding shapes the course of remedial measures.

Understanding elements—their defining attributes and manifestations in human life—is essential for understanding the Ayurvedic way of life.

Elements - The building blocks of matter

Ayurveda believes that every material existence—living or non-living—comprises five fundamental elements: ether (space), air, fire, water, and earth. These elements combine in varying proportions to fill the universe with such diversity. Stars, planets, oceans, rivers, trees, rocks, animals, microorganisms, and various life forms combine one or more of these elements.

Human beings are also made up of elements, but there is one notable difference between living and non-living. While one or more elements can form material objects, all five elements must come together to create life. Even if one element is missing, life cannot exist. Moreover, elements always form a unique composition to create a new life, so no two humans have the same combination.

How elements relate to the body and mind

Elements are also the building blocks of tissues and organs in each cell. But Ayurvedic elements should not be understood as physical presences in the body. They are more like ideas that cannot be measured but can only be identified.

Each element has distinct qualities or attributes reflected in an individual's mind-body makeup. For example, fire can be observed in the strength of human will. Water is found in the blood, saliva, and bodily fluids. Likewise, the presence of all elements can be observed by paying close attention to your body, mind, emotions, and sensations.

In human beings, elements combine to form three life energies collectively known as doshas. Unlike elements, which are not literal in their meaning but have a deeper significance, doshas are measurable forces that govern various physiological functions, like digestion, tissue building, blood circulation, neural coordination, etc.

Ether (space)

Ether or space is the first and subtlest element that makes up a major part (99%) of the universe. It represents emptiness, i.e., the absence of other elements. It is the unoccupied space that creates room for other elements to fill. Ether is inherently present in all five elements, as everything originates from it. It is omnipresent, expansive, and knows no boundaries. In Sanskrit, the ether element is called *Akasha*, meaning the sky, which signifies its endless character.

The unbound character of the human mind is the psychological manifestation of ether. Our ideas, imaginations, aspirations, thoughts, and creative abilities are limitless because we are powered by ether. The mind needs no medium to travel and can move seamlessly through space and time.

In the body, the physical presence of ether can be recognized in the lungs, blood vessels, between the intestines, deep inside ears, nasal cavities, and at the center of bones. Ether is perceived through the sense of hearing. Its sensory organ is the ear, and the mouth is the organ of action.

Qualities and significance

Ether has no attributes of its own and is identified by a lack of other elemental qualities. It is cool because it lacks fire's warmth; it is dry because it does not have the soothing influence of water; it is light and formless because it lacks the groundedness of earth; it is immobile because it lacks air movement. Ether element also symbolizes the soul due to its lack of physical form.

Ether is a destructive force and must be filled with other elements. The other four elements act as a container for limiting its vastness. For example, food made from other elements is needed to fill up the intestines; otherwise, the body will not be able to function. Too much space inside the body can deform structures and cause cell death. Lungs have no use except when filled with air. Emptiness in life can disturb peace of mind if not superseded by love (nourishment) and fulfilling pursuits.

Functions of the ether element

The primary function of the ether element is to provide space for organs and tissues. When in balance, your muscles have enough space for contraction and expansion. You feel carefree and have a sense of deep connection with the divine.

When the ether goes out of balance, it can cause hearing problems or tissue deformation. Abnormal bodily sounds, like cracking of joints, wheezing, or a sudden change in voice, may indicate an imbalance. Having less ether can also create problems.

The following symptoms can identify an imbalance in the ether:

- Extreme carelessness or a sense of detachment
- Parkinson's disease (due to the destruction of brain cells)
- Speech or hearing disorders
- Thyroid problems
- Stubbornness
- Sore muscles
- Stiff joints
- Insomnia and other sleep-related issues

Air

Air—the primary force behind life on this planet—is the second most subtle element of Ayurveda. It is the first element to originate from the ether and takes the space created by it. Air represents kinetic energy that enables all kinds of movement and communication.

The physical manifestation of air can be observed in all those biological processes that require mobility and exchange. Breathing, movement of food inside the intestines, blood flow, transfer of nutrients, toxin elimination, and nervous coordination represent the presence of air.

The mental manifestation of air can be recognized in the mind's flow of thoughts and fluidity. Air is perceived through the sense of touch. Its sensory organ is the skin, and hands are the organ of action.

Qualities and significance

Cool, dry, rough, irregular, light, and mobile qualities characterize air. It imparts these very attributes to the human body and mind. Our thoughts and emotions can be irregular and fluctuating. Dry and rough skin, periods of indiscipline, uncertainty in mind, difficulty in making decisions, and changing inclinations are all expressions of the air element.

In Ayurveda, the air is considered the primordial energy of the universe and the giver of *prana* (the vital energy of life). Control over this element is considered essential for living life to its fullest. If air moves too fast in the system, it can bring hyperactivity in thoughts and actions. On the other hand, too slow movement can result in a sluggish mind, improper detoxification, or poor blood circulation.

Controlling the air element by consciously directing the breath is one of the most important aspects of Ayurvedic healing. The quality of your breath determines your vitality and enthusiasm for life, the health of your tissues, and your ability to cope with daily challenges. Pranayama yoga practices aim to maximize the prana energy and enable an optimal flow of air.

Functions of the air element

Air fills the space created by ether and fuels the fire. The body's primary function is facilitating communication between the brain and other organs. When you have the right amount of air in your system, you are able to think clearly and feel creatively stimulated. Balance in the air element is also vital for the optimal functioning of sensory organs, proper blood **circulation**, bowel regularity, and detoxification.

When the air element is deficient or in excess, it may cause the following problems:

- Respiratory disorders
- Scattered and foggy mind
- Sleeplessness
- Constipation or diarrhea
- Abdominal bloating and pain
- Either fatigued or hyperactive
- Mental fatigue
- Dry skin and hair
- Irregular heartbeat
- Frequent joint or muscle pain
- Severe menstrual cramps

Fire

Fire is the third element of Ayurveda that represents the powerful force of transformation. It comes after ether and air and contains the essence of both elements within it. Ether provides the space for it to burn, and air gives it the strength to go on and facilitates it's working.

All kinds of metabolic reactions and biochemical changes inside the body can be seen as an expression of fire. The breakdown of food by digestive juices, carbs conversion into glucose, nutrients assimilation into tissues, hormonal secretion, blood glucose maintenance, and enzymatic reactions are all physical manifestations of the fire element.

Its agents are bile juices, enzymes, neurochemicals, red blood cells, and various hormones. Without fire, our food will not convert into energy, and there will be no hormones to make us feel emotions.

The mental manifestation of fire can be observed in how we process raw information and assimilate it into permanent memory. Its transformative quality is also expressed in the strength of human will, intellectual traits of the mind, the force of our character, passionate emotions, and the desire for power. Fire is associated with the sense of vision and direction, and its primary organs are the eyes (sensory) and feet (action).

Qualities and significance

Fire is characterized by hot, sharp, light, intense, clear, and penetrating qualities. In Ayurvedic philosophy, fire (*agni*) energy is also known as the digestive flame, which provides the body the fuel to go on. It is the primary metabolic force that enables us to digest food and newly acquired information and experiences of our worldly life. It helps us convert ideas into action. In other words, fire connects us to the outer world. If the fire is disturbed, our connection with the outside world may suffer.

However, this also means that all incoming factors, whether in the form of food or experiences, have the potential to disturb this element. Since digestion is recognized as the most important aspect of overall wellness and the root cause of all diseases, optimal strength of fire is seen as a precondition for leading a healthy and productive life.

Therefore, controlling fire through conscious eating (of food and ideas) is considered crucial for a healthy body-mind. If left unrestrained, fire can become destructive and burn everything. In living beings, it is always accompanied by water—the soothing force of nature that has the power to confine the fire element.

Functions of the fire element

The primary functions of fire are to facilitate digestion and metabolism, provide energy, manage hormonal actions, produce sweat, and keep us warm. When in balance, it provides sharpness of vision, intellect, focus, and confidence. The right amount of fire in your system is vital for healthy digestion and nutrient absorption.

When the fire goes out of balance, it can cause the following symptoms:

- Anxiety and fear
- Excessive thirst and hunger
- Self-criticism
- Lusterless skin and hair
- Low energy
- Frequent digestive problems
- Lacking enthusiasm in the morning
- Being frequently angry or snappy at others
- Sleeplessness and excessive dreaming
- Hyperactive and over-competitive mind

- Recurring skin problems like acne, rashes, and boils
- Mouth sores

Water

Water—the fourth (second heaviest) element of Ayurveda—represents nature's nourishing, soothing side that sustains life. It is the most abundant element on the earth's surface, making up about 60% of the human body.

The physical manifestations of water can be recognized in lymphatic fluids, mucous membranes, saliva, reproductive fluids, and blood. It regulates the body temperature, lubricates joints for smooth movement, removes metabolic waste, soothes inflammation and pain, keeps the skin hydrated, and facilitates the nervous system.

Its psychological manifestation can be observed in emotional qualities like empathy, contentment, compassion, love, friendship, devotion, loyalty, support, kindness, and warmth toward others. Water is perceived through the sense of taste. Its sensory organ is the tongue, and the urethra is the organ of action.

Qualities and significance

Water is characterized by cool, moist, nourishing, smooth, soft, flowing, and moving qualities. It protects us from the harshness of other elements and provides a medium of cohesion to keep them all together. It fills the space created by ether, hydrates, and protects against the dryness of the air, pacifies the fire's heat, and enables the earth to hold its form.

Water plays a profound role in healing and nourishment. It represents life's vital fluid, giving longevity and immunity against disorders. But having too much of it is not desirable, as water can dilute the strength of fire.

Functions of the water element

The most important function of water is to keep your brain healthy and energized. In addition, it facilitates detoxification, maintains a steady body temperature, produces mucus, aids digestion, boosts nutrient utilization, and enhances physical and mental stamina. It also helps lower inflammation and protects against chronic conditions like arthritis and heart problems. When maintained in equilibrium, water has the ability to heal and slow down the degeneration associated with aging.

A deficiency in the water element is easily noticeable. It can cause dehydration, dry skin, a sluggish mind, weak reproductive organs, and an accumulation of toxins. Having excess water can make other elements more dominant—and hence more destructive since water is the protector.

This soothing energy can cause the following symptoms when it goes out of balance:

- Water retention
- Swollen feet and ankles
- Puffy face and eyes
- Joint and muscle stiffness
- Low muscle endurance/getting tired easily
- Difficulty concentrating
- Heavy menstruation
- Sluggish digestion and bloating
- Loss of appetite
- Feeling depressed or low most of the time

- Lethargy and physical fatigue
- Nasal or sinus congestion
- Dry and rough skin

Earth

Earth is the heaviest element that symbolizes the grounded nature of life. The solid form of matter gives the universe its physical existence, enabling other elements to work within. Earth also restrains other elements and prevents them from turning destructive. Without the boundaries of the earth, ether will fill the universe, and there will be no existence of matter. It is the earth that limits the expanse of ether, pacifies the fire, grounds the movement of air, and holds the flow of water within itself.

Earth combines with water to form bones, muscles, cartilage, tendons, joints, tissues, fats, skin, hair, and all organs in the body. Its physical manifestation is the very frame and structure of the body. Earth is perceived through the sense of smell. Its associated organs are the nose (sensory) and rectum (action).

The mental manifestation of earth can be recognized in emotional qualities like calmness, humility, discipline, regularity, empathy, faith, honesty, gratitude, groundedness, and a tendency to seek stability in life.

Qualities and significance

Earth is characterized by cool, dry, rough, stable, heavy, calm, hard, and dense qualities. Every material existence that has a physical form is composed of earth. The food we eat is also an expression of the earth, which means it enters the body with every meal. This makes this element highly prone to imbalance.

Earth holds the key to both health and disease. An excess of this element (when we eat more than we burn) can make us vulnerable to lifestyle disorders like obesity and heart problems. On the other hand, its deficiency can weaken bones and reduce muscle mass. Nutrition and physical exercise are extremely important factors for maintaining an optimal balance of this element.

Functions of the earth

The primary function of the earth is to build and repair—and bring us closer to who we are. When you have a strong presence of the earth in your system, you feel deeply connected and in full control of your feelings, thoughts, emotions, and expectations. Earth also grants well-formed and strong musculature, robust bones, smooth and healthy skin, and excellent stamina. During pregnancy, a strong presence of the earth (from nutrient-dense foods) is desirable as it helps form a healthy fetus.

Lack of proper nutrition, unhealthy eating habits, and a sedentary lifestyle can throw this element out of balance. The following signs may indicate an imbalance:

- Excess weight gain
- Osteoporosis
- Frequent muscle injuries
- Frequent infections and allergies
- Episodes of heavy-heartedness
- Being extremely afraid of change
- Lack of motivation
- Chronic constipation
- Feeling hopeless and depressed

- Oversleeping or difficulty getting up in the morning
- Laziness

Elements: Senses, organs, and functions

Elements	Senses	Sensory organ	Organ of action	Function
Ether	Sound	Ear	Mouth and vocal cords	Speaking
Air	Touch	Skin	Hands	Grasping
Fire	Sight	Eyes	Feet	Moving
Water	Taste	Tongue	Genitals	Procreating
Earth	Smell	Nose	Rectum	Excreting or eliminating

Elements are closely interlinked together

It is important to note that elements are not separate entities. They work in close cooperation and coordination with each other, and perfect harmony between them is essential for proper functioning. One element's imbalance (deficiency or excess) can also affect the other. Remedying one problem will not improve the condition unless the natural balance is restored.

For example, if you have a low digestive fire, taking super-nourishing foods may not help much, as your food will not get digested properly. Good digestive strength and nutrition will not help much if the circulation is poor, or you do not drink sufficient water.

The Ayurvedic way of life takes a holistic view of disease (imbalance). It proposes a multipronged lifestyle aimed at restoring and maintaining a perfect balance between all five elements while also considering a person's constitution.

Chapter 3

Doshas

What are doshas?

Ayurveda believes that the nature of this universe is cyclical. Everything passes through three phases—manifestation, existence, and destruction—and the cycle of birth and rebirth continues. Nothing new is ever created. Things only transition from one phase to another.

Years, seasons, days, the sun, the moon, and even living beings follow the same cyclical pattern of creation, action, and restoration. Nature has a season of full bloom (spring), a time for action (summer), and then a gradual retreat to hibernation (fall/winter).

According to Ayurveda, three primordial energies keep the cycle in motion: the anabolic energy that builds (Kapha), the metabolic energy that sustains (Pitta), and finally, the catabolic energy that breaks things down to their original state and makes room for a new beginning (Vata).

Since the microcosm only reflects the macrocosm, these energies are also found inside plants, animals, humans, and everything created in the universe. Together, three life forces carry out their respective functions of building tissues, sustaining life processes, and releasing energy. In the context of health and Ayurvedic medicine, they are referred to as 'doshas.'

Five elements make three doshas

Elements from nature combine to form the three doshas. Space and air combine to create Vata, the energy of movement and transportation; fire and water unite to form the transformative metabolic energy of Pitta; earth and water coalesce to form the cohesive force of Kapha.

Doshas collectively govern various physiological and psychological functions necessary to support life. Just like elements, they also form a unique composition every time to create a new life and are invariably present in everything that *lives*. But doshas should not be viewed as a static presence in the body. They are dynamic forces always working and changing, each constantly affecting and being affected by present environmental conditions.

Each dosha is characterized by a unique set of qualities that represents the combined features of its elements. While they are mutually dependent and work in cooperation, each energy is responsible for carrying out different functions and imparts a distinct character to an individual's temperament.

Vata

Vata is a union of air and ether elements. It is the ruling force behind all kinds of movement, transportation, and communication in the body. Respiration, blood circulation, transfer of nutrients, movement of food through the digestive tract, waste elimination, working of the five senses, the central nervous system, neural impulses, coordination between the brain and other organs, and all physiological functions that require mobility are performed by Vata dosha.

Think of Vata as currents inside the body, without which one part of the body cannot connect with the other. And since organs are interdependent, the whole system will fail. Without it, the heart will not be able to pump blood, the lungs will not breathe, and the brain will have no control over muscles.

The functions of Vata are catabolic in nature. It breaks down things and releases energy. It governs basic cellular functions like how cells divide and how respiration breaks down sugar into smaller molecules.

In the Ayurvedic clock, Vata comes at the end of the day, end of the year (fall and winter), and end of digestion (excretion). It is dominant early in the morning between 2 a.m. and 6 a.m. and in the afternoon between 2 p.m. and 6 p.m. It also becomes prominent in the later years of human life. Older adults are at a greater risk of Vata-related health problems.

Qualities and significance

Vata is creative, imaginative, vivacious, enthusiastic, and ever-changing. On a cosmic level, Purusha (consciousness or soul) and Prakriti (matter) merge because of *Prana*, which is the subtle essence of Vata.

The primary site of Vata inside the body is the colon, with the waist, thighs, ears, bones, and skin being closely related. It is responsible for the initiation and execution of natural urges like eating or urinating. Vata is associated with the astringent taste within Ayurveda's Shad Rasa (six tastes), and its seasons are autumn and winter.

Subdoshas of Vata: Functions, locations, and signs of imbalance

Each Ayurvedic dosha is further divided into five sub-categories known as Subdoshas, which govern specific functions, organs, and emotions.

Sub dosha	Location	Function	Action	Signs of disturbance
Prana	Heart, throat, head, respiratory organs, and brain	Movement of air, food, and water from outside to the body	Inhalation and perception through the senses	Anxiety, insomnia, asthma
Udana	Chest, lung, and naval	Movement from the body to the outside	Speech, self-expression, enthusiasm and exhalation	Acid reflux, stuttering
Samana	Stomach and small intestine	Movement from the periphery to the center	Manages peristaltic movement of the digestive system	Impaired digestion

Vyana	Center of the heart	Movement from the center to the periphery	Manages Musculo skeletal movement and blood circulation	Hyperten-sion, arrhythmia, tremor, panic
Apana	Colon and the anus	Downward impulses	Defecation, urination, menstrua-tion, sexual discharges, and childbirth	Constipa-tion, menstrual disorders, or genito-urinary problems

Pitta

Pitta is the combined energy of fire and water elements. Where there is fire, there has to be water; otherwise, the fire will burn everything. When these two elements merge, they form a transformative force capable of sustaining life. Pitta governs all kinds of metabolic reactions and biochemical changes.

It is responsible for breaking down food, releasing enzymes and digestive juices, converting macronutrients to simpler molecules (like glucose and amino acids), and assimilating nutrients into tissues. Pitta is also responsible for producing, releasing, storing, and maintaining an ideal balance of hormones. Since it is heavily involved in the endocrine system, it controls how we feel and act.

Pitta is the metabolic energy that supplies the fuel for action. It is required for digesting foods as well as ideas. It breaks down, analyses, understands, organizes, and then assimilates all the incoming information and experiences. It is Pitta that transforms our thoughts into intelligence and intelligence into pure awareness. Anything that needs to be processed or converted from one form to another is the function of Pitta dosha.

Qualities and significance

Pitta is derived from the Sanskrit word 'tapa,' which means heat, concentration, or austerity. It represents heat and intensity in the mind, body, and spirit. On a cosmic level, Pitta is related to the radiant energy of Surya (the sun) and Buddhi (the universal intelligence). If this sounds like fire (agni), it is because the two are inherent to each other's existence. Pitta is the container, and agni is the content.

Pitta is found in every body cell as Tejas, the cellular intelligence and the subtlest essence of this dosha. It produces hunger, thirst, appetite, complexion, intelligence, courage, valor, and softness of the skin tissues. The main location of Pitta is the navel and small intestines. Still, it also resides in subcutaneous fat, the grey matter of the brain, stomach, sweat, blood, eyes, and, specifically, the liver, spleen, and gallbladder.

Pitta dominates a major part of active human life. In the Ayurvedic clock, it comes in the middle: middle of the year (the summer season), middle of the day, and middle of the night. It is dominant from 10 a.m. to 2 p.m. in the daytime and from 10 p.m. to 2 a.m. at night.

Subdoshas of Pitta: Functions, locations, and signs of imbalance

Sub doshas	Location	Functions	Action	Signs of disturbance
Pachak	Lower stomach and small intestine	Initial digestion of food	Digestion and metabolism	Hyperacidity, accumulation of ama
Ranjak	Liver, gallbladder, and spleen	Formation of red blood cells and secondary tissues	Gives color to blood and stool	Liver disorders, anemia
Sadhak	Heart and brain	Conversion of knowledge and control of higher mental functions	Digest thoughts and ideas	Confusion, anger, foggy mind
Alochak	Eyes	Perception of knowledge	Visual perception	Eye problems
Bhrajak	Skin	Complexion and luster of the skin	Temperature and skin pigmentation	Rashes, acne breakouts

Kapha

Kapha is the amalgamation of earth and water elements. It is the anabolic energy of life that builds the physical form of the body. The primary function of Kapha is to oversee all kinds of cohesion and lubrication inside the body. Think of Kapha as a glue that holds together bones, muscles, fats, tissues, and joints.

It adds density to bones and joints, builds cells, and tissues, and provides enough lubrication (mucus) for their smooth functioning.

Kapha is heavily involved in immune functions and wound healing, producing new cells to replace dead ones. This includes the production of immune cells. It also keeps inflammation in check and slows down the aging process.

Qualities and significance

Kapha is a cosmic representation of the moon or the 'soma.' It is cool, white, feminine, healing, and nourishing. It embodies the love and warmth of a mother and is best exemplified by breast milk. Kapha's molecules hug each other, creating a dense mass, hence the term "to hug."

Kapha is akin to a person's formative years, which is considered the first 16 years of life. It is dominant in the early morning (from 6 a.m. to 10 a.m.), the early evening (from 6 p.m. to 10 p.m.), and the late winter and spring seasons. It is closely related to the sweet and salty tastes of Shad Rasa.

Kapha is primarily located in the stomach, but it also guides the functions of the GI tract and lungs (its main therapeutic site). Kapha can be seen in the brain and the white matter, the myelin sheath, cerebrospinal fluid, and the synovial fluid of joints. Towards the later stage of life, the protective force of Kapha takes backstage, and Vata becomes more and more dominant. This increases the risk of developing inflammatory conditions like rheumatoid arthritis.

Subdoshas of Kapha: Functions, locations, and signs of imbalance

Sub doshas	Location	Function	Action	Signs of disturbance
Kledak	The upper part of the stomach	Stomach lubrication	Moistens and liquefies foods in the initial stage of digestion	Indigestion
Avalam-bak	Heart, chest, and lung	Supports the heart and low back	Lubricates the heart and lungs	Heart, lung, or spine disorders
Bodhak	Mouth, tongue, and throat	Protection of mucous membrane of mouth and perception of taste	Lubricates mouth and the throat	Hoarse voice
Tarpak	Head, sinuses, and cerebros-pinal fluid	Nourishes the sense and motor organs	Protects the brain and spinal cord from external shocks	Brain fog, headache, sinus congestion
Shleshak	Joints	Lubricates the joints	Lubricates the joints	Arthritis, edema

How doshas influence health and disease

Dosha translates from Sanskrit as "the faulty one" or "the one prone to corruption." This means that while these energies are vital for life, they often go out of balance.

In normal times, when doshas work in harmony, they support a healthy and disease-free life. But when this equilibrium is disturbed—either due to environmental conditions or poor lifestyle choices—one or more of them may go out of balance.

An imbalance of dosha refers to an over-accumulation of energy, which may happen when its corresponding elements are in excess. For example, hot weather represents a dominating fire element, which can increase the Pitta dosha if not countered with lots of water-rich and cooling foods. Similarly, a lack of routine can bring restlessness and increase Vata in the body.

When these life-giving forces increase or decrease out of proportion, they acquire a destructive nature and start affecting every aspect of well-being, from skin texture and mood to sleep and digestion. The imbalance of doshas is considered the root cause of all diseases in Ayurvedic philosophy. In fact, this is the foundation on which Ayurvedic medicine works. Ayurveda views disease as an imbalance of some dosha and prescribes correcting measures like foods, herbs, medicines, therapies, and yoga—all targeted toward restoring balance.

Each dosha is responsible for causing different kinds of health problems. And since they are mutually dependent on each other, an imbalance in one may also influence the working of others. For example, frequent digestive problems do not necessarily indicate Pitta imbalance. It can also happen due to sluggish movement of food inside the digestive tract or excessive dryness, which are Vata-related problems. An accumulation of Kapha inside the colon can also cause congestion and clogging.

An Ayurvedic practitioner can make the correct diagnosis by looking at all the physical and emotional symptoms combined.

Vata and health

Vata's defining attributes are the same as air and space: cool, light, dry, rough, mobile, clear, and irregular. An excess of any of these qualities can throw it out of balance. Certain factors such as dry and windy weather, consumption of canned and frozen foods, lack of discipline, irregular sleep patterns, and lack of routine can amplify imbalances in the body. Conversely, conditions like warmth, nourishment, stability, moisture, discipline, and relaxation can help restore balance. To achieve a Vata-pacifying lifestyle, restorative yoga poses, and deep breathing exercises play a crucial role.

When in balance

When Vata works properly, it provides clear senses, clarity of thought and expression, congestion-free breathing, enhanced flow of blood and nutrients, complete and consistent elimination, and original thinking. It is also the driving force behind creative expressions, such as art and innovation.

Signs of Vata imbalance

When out of balance, Vata may cause constipation (irregular or incomplete elimination), intestinal bloating, flatulence, dry skin and hair, poor blood circulation, low stamina, breathing difficulties, restlessness, hyperactivity, anxious mind, scattered thoughts, impaired speech, a lapse in memory, and cognitive difficulties. Poor circulation may also cause joint and muscle pain. A hyperactive and restless mind can make it difficult to fall asleep, increasing stress levels.

Pitta and health

The qualities of Pitta are similar to that of firewater (acid and bile). It is hot, sharp, penetrating, light, mobile, and oily. An excess of these qualities can cause an imbalance of Pitta. For example, oily and spicy foods, hot weather, or excessive workload (burnout) may increase Pitta dosha. Opposite qualities like a cool environment, windy weather, fresh fruits and vegetables, drinking loads of water, calming yoga poses, and relaxation practices like aromatherapy can help bring it back to balance.

When in balance

When Pitta is in proportion, it gives a hearty appetite, speedy metabolism, excellent eyesight, intense emotions, radiant skin and hair, a focused and motivated mind, sharp intellect, and balanced hormones. For women, it means regular and less painful periods.

Ensuring a well-maintained balance of the Pitta dosha can significantly contribute to the overall well-being of women as they encounter different stages of life and undergo hormonal changes. Whether during menstruation, childbirth, or menopause, striving for this balance can assist women in feeling their best and aid in a smoother transition throughout these phases.

Signs of Pitta imbalance

When out of balance, Pitta starts producing excess digestive juices, hormones, and enzymes that can cause diarrhea, heartburn, acid reflux, ulcers, acne, rashes, boils, mood swings, bleeding disorders, and inflammation. Women may experience heavy and painful PMS, PCOD, or irregular cycles. The skin and hair start producing too much oil. Hormonal imbalances also interfere with sleep, and one may experience frequent dream interruptions at night. Passionate emotions like anger and jealousy may become too intense.

Kapha and health

Kapha's defining attributes are slimy, sticky, slow, dull, moist, oily, dense, heavy, cool, and stable. An excess of these qualities can make it go out of balance and affect health in multiple ways. The opposite qualities of warm, light, dry, and stimulating can help it regain balance. For example, lack of physical activity (dull) and too much food (heavy) can increase Kapha and lead to weight gain. On the other hand, physical exercise, stimulating yoga poses, and light meals can help restore balance.

When in balance

When Kapha is in proportion, it provides strong tissues and joints, robust stamina, soft and smooth skin, well-nourished hair, emotional stability, peaceful sleep, and healthy immune function. It also ensures sexual and reproductive well-being.

Signs of Kapha imbalance

When Kapha goes out of proportion, it starts producing too much mucus. As a result, you may experience sinus infections, lung congestion, and allergies. If the imbalance is not corrected in time, it can also cause chronic problems like water retention, weight gain, obesity, and even diabetes and cardiovascular diseases. Its stable nature can quickly take the form of stubbornness, laziness, and arrogance.

It can cause over sleepiness, making it increasingly difficult to get up in the morning. Kapha imbalance is also believed to cause many serious mental disorders like heavy-heartedness and various forms of depression.

Chapter 4

Prakriti (Constitution): Ayurvedic Body-Mind Types

C elebrating diversity while also appreciating individuality is the essence of Ayurvedic healing. This ancient philosophy recognizes that each person is unique and needs specialized care tailored to their personality. Moreover, this specialized care must come from within and not depend too much on remedial measures.

Ayurveda believes that every person needs to take charge of their own health and consciously choose a lifestyle that appreciates their uniqueness. Understanding who you are—the physical body and the energy within—is essential for fully appreciating yourself and will ultimately bring empowerment.

Prakriti - The composition of different doshas

Many people wonder about the vast range of differences among human beings. Although we are all made up of the same materials and function in a similar physiological manner, our responses to life vary tremendously.

One medicine may completely heal one person and still prove ineffective for another person of the same age, sex, height, weight, body-mass index, and medical preconditions. The same ayurvedic medicine may heal two people but does not necessarily exhibit the same potency. Some people are vulnerable to particular food or weather, while others seem unaffected. Some people can manage to stay in shape with little effort, whereas others find it extremely difficult to lose a few pounds.

Human beings also exhibit great diversity in emotional intelligence and mental aptitude. So, what makes people so different in their adaptability to the environment's demands? Why can some people handle setbacks in life better than others? Why is one person's food another person's poison?

All these questions can be answered by simply understanding that each person is born with a unique composition of doshas, known as their Ayurvedic constitution or Prakriti. This unique bio-genomic makeup is responsible for a person's unique set of qualities, personality traits, body structure, temperament, inclinations, and vulnerabilities in life.

The three doshas are present in everyone but rarely in equal quantities. More often than not, one (or more than one) dosha is more proportionate than others. The dominating dosha contributes more to the individual's mind-body makeup and is responsible for most (but not all) of their physical, mental, and emotional qualities.

Assessment of Prakriti

The assessment of Prakriti combines both direct and indirect means. The direct method involves physically examining body temperature, frame and structure, skin texture and oiliness, and pulse rate. A thorough understanding is attained by the indirect method.

In order to find the dominant dosha, an individual's personality is assessed on a few questions related to their lifestyle, such as appetite, sleep pattern, bowel routine, anger response, mental disposition, skin and hair type, recurring health problems, and other lifetime tendencies. Based on how far their personal attributes relate to each dosha, the relative dosha proportion is identified.

Benefits of knowing your dominant dosha

The dominating dosha is responsible for a person's general quality of life. It determines their reaction to foods, environmental conditions, and their response to therapies. Most importantly, it helps determine their risks and vulnerabilities to external stimuli, which can help prevent imbalances beforehand. For example, if a person is Pitta-dominant, they have a greater risk of imbalance in the summer when Pitta is naturally high. This knowledge can help them make lifestyle adjustments and avoid triggers.

Knowing your dosha type can also help you design your personalized self-care regimen. It can help you choose the right skincare products, eat the right foods at the proper time, get the right herbal supplements, practice the right yoga poses, and meditate at the right time.

The benefits of knowing your constitution are:

- Prevention of imbalance
- Personalized self-care
- Prognosis of diseases
- Selection of appropriate skin products
- Selection of appropriate treatment
- Selection of appropriate rejuvenation therapy

The difference between Prakriti and Vikriti

Prakriti (original creation)

The Prakriti of a person is determined at the time of birth and stays the same throughout life. Apart from the dominating dosha of the father and mother, four factors play a major role in forming a constitution.

- The intention of parents at the time of conception
- The heredity of parents
- The diet and lifestyle of the mother during pregnancy
- The conditions prevalent in the womb, cervix, and vagina during pregnancy and at the time of birth

Vikriti (after creation)

Vikriti refers to the current imbalance a person might be having. It can be due to improper diet, neglect, unhealthy practices, environmental conditions, or poor lifestyle choices.

The dominating dosha should not be understood as an accumulation or excess, although it is in higher proportion than others. For example, high Pitta is normal for a Pitta-dominant person but may cause health problems in some other Prakriti. But if the same person experiences a further increase in Pitta dosha, it is called an imbalance or Vikriti.

Prakriti is our nature, whereas Vikriti is our current state. Vikriti must be corrected by making appropriate lifestyle adjustments or taking proper medications. Both Prakriti and Vikriti are taken into consideration for diagnosing diseases, as well as for recommending treatments.

Ayurvedic body types

Based on the dominant dosha type, Ayurveda recognizes seven types of Prakriti.

1. Vata-dominant
2. Pitta-dominant
3. Kapha-dominant
4. Vata-Pitta
5. Pitta-Kapha
6. Vata-Kapha
7. Vata-Pitta-Kapha

Vata-dominant mind-body type

Physical characteristics

Individuals of Vata-dominant body type have a lot of air and space in their constitution, which accounts for their narrow body frame, small structure, and delicate musculature. They have a slightly colder body temperature than people of other doshas, and they naturally prefer warm and moist climates. Their skin and hair texture resembles the qualities of air and space, i.e., dry, dull, rough, and brittle.

Vata-dominant people have an average appetite, metabolism, and lifespan—which lies somewhere between Pitta and Kapha. They age neither too slowly nor too fast. This dosha's light, quick, moving qualities ensure a slim build and high energy for these body types, and they are usually very brisk in both physical and mental activities.

Furthermore, they prefer an active lifestyle and generally find it hard to gain muscle mass. True to their agile nature, Vata individuals are also light sleepers and prefer to sleep for fewer hours than other ayurvedic body types.

However, Vata cannot have fixed rules because this dosha is inherently erratic and irregular. The ether element does not respect rules. It can make small and narrow frames and athletic body types. This is the most striking feature of Vata Prakriti. Its irregular quality makes it very difficult to assess the correct dosha type.

Mental and emotional qualities

Vata is the energy responsible for cognitive functions, and it naturally makes creative minds and original thinkers. Individuals of this mind-body type are capable of thinking out of the box; they can see connections that no one else can. Their senses are quick and clear, and they are always willing to try and learn new skills. Also, having quick grasping power, Vata can quickly and easily learn new things. However, they usually have poor long-term memory, which may negate some of the benefits of their exceptional learning skills.

Because of their ruling air element, Vata-dominant individuals are full of life (*Prana*). They are vivacious, easy-going, light-spirited, quick-witted, enthusiastic, and excellent communicators. Their temperament is composed, and they have a fairly decent amount of control over their anger, though not as much as Kapha. Their preferences in life are also symbolic of the air—they like to travel and explore new things.

Both air and ether elements are unbound by their very nature, and this quality is also seen in people governed by this dosha.

Vata-minded individuals value freedom most of all. They like to work in their own flow rather than being dictated to by premade rules and conditions. However, this also means they can easily lose direction if their flow is unrestricted by discipline and routine.

The temperament of Vata-dominant people can sometimes be like air—moving and unstable. They easily get bored and lose interest in things they once started with so much enthusiasm. They are generally inclined towards an adventurous life and do not like to settle on one thing for too long.

Tendencies and vulnerabilities

Vata individuals usually have poor general immunity against common infections. Because of the uncertain nature of this dosha, they face all kinds of irregularities in their day-to-day life: irregular appetite, fluctuating mood, erratic sleep, irregular menstruation, irregular bowel movements, alternating constipation, and diarrhea, and alternating opposite conditions. Constipation can be a recurring and extremely common problem.

Vata Prakriti shows a general intolerance towards cold and windy weather, spicy foods, and cooling herbs. During winter and autumn, they find it increasingly difficult to hydrate their skin.

The general tendency to engage in excessive physical activity can make Vata vulnerable to anxiety, stress, restlessness, and insomnia. Their lifelong vulnerability is to allergies, lung diseases, and respiratory disorders. In old age, they are susceptible to developing neurological conditions characterized by memory loss and cognitive decline, such as dementia.

Vata attributes and manifestations

Attributes of Vata	Physical and mental manifestations
Light	Thin and small frame, delicate muscles, less muscle mass, and light body weight
Rough	Cracked skin and nails, stiff joints, and brittle hair
Dry	Dry skin, lips, tongue, eyes, scalp, and internal organs (constipation)
Mobile	Brisk walking, fast speech, frequent travel, multitasking, and a scattered and unstable mind
Erratic	Irregular eating, sleeping, and lifestyle
Cold	Cold hands and feet, poor circulation
Subtle	Fear, anxiety, insecurity, and mood swings

Prevention of imbalance

Vata imbalance can be prevented by avoiding aggravating factors, such as refrigerated foods, cold and windy weather, drying and cooling herbs, spicy meals, raw vegetables, and carbonated beverages.

Vata is innately erratic and very prone to disorders. Discipline is vital for keeping this dosha in check. It is important to make a schedule for everything. Try to plan and organize your life at every level, from sleep and meals to work. Going to bed at the same time every day, eating at regular intervals, planning your meals, writing a journal, and even settling a daily time for bowel movements can greatly improve your overall quality of life.

People of Vata dosha benefit from a nourishing, hearty diet with plenty of protein and whole grains. It is also important to consume high-quality fats like ghee and olive oil to prevent dryness of internal organs. However, make sure always to eat warm and well-cooked food.

Also, try to consume water and fluids at room temperature. Cold water and iced drinks can harm digestive fire. And since this dosha already has a low agni, it can contribute to digestive problems like constipation and bloating. Vata individuals should strictly avoid skipping meals, as it can increase ether element and harm agni.

Vata skin can benefit from heavy-duty moisturizers and oils like sesame, almond, shea butter, or mustard oil. Coconut oil and aloe vera are great moisturizers, but their cooling potency can worsen skin problems for Vata. If you like aloe vera, look for moisturizers with other warming and balancing ingredients.

Pitta-dominant mind-body type

Physical characteristics

Individuals with Pitta-dominant Prakriti have a medium frame and average musculature. Their bones and muscles are fairly strong—not as robust as Kapha but stronger than Vata. Because their constitution has more fire than other doshas, their body temperature is noticeably warmer. The texture of their skin and hair signifies the oily quality of Pitta and is mostly on the greasier side.

Pitta is the ruling energy of metabolism, which is reflected in this dosha type's remarkable digestive strength and appetite. Their food and water consumption are naturally higher than other Ayurvedic body types, yet they do not gain too much weight because of a high basal metabolic rate. Individuals with a Pitta body type have the ability to lose or gain weight as desired easily. However, their quick metabolism can also lead to increased free radicals and faster aging, resulting in premature wrinkles and hair greying. In terms of general immunity and sleep quality, Pitta falls somewhere between Vata and Kapha.

Mental and emotional qualities

Pitta dosha makes sharp, fiery, focused, highly motivated, and strong-willed personalities. These individuals may not be as creative as Vata, but they are resourceful and great at implementing ideas. The powerful element of fire gives them a remarkably sharp intellect and high information processing speed, enabling them to organize and digest ideas beautifully.

Pitta's passion and dedication are exemplary; once they have set their heart on something, they will stop at nothing to achieve that goal. Their temperament signifies the intensity of their ruling element, and they generally display strong emotions in love and relationships.

Tendencies and vulnerabilities

Pitta-dominant individuals tend to overthink and overwork. Their tendency to take up more work than they can reasonably handle can make them vulnerable to stress and sleep loss. Their overactive minds can also make their sleep fragmented and irregular.

Also, a general tendency to seek perfection in everything can make them obsess excessively over simple tasks. Sometimes, they immerse themselves so much in work that they forget to sleep or eat. Because of Pitta's high food and water needs, missing meals can easily make them irritable and fatigued.

Pitta people prefer cold and windy conditions and are generally intolerant of hot and humid weather. In the summer season, their skin can start producing too much sebum, and their digestion can go from robust to delicate. Skin problems like acne, blisters, rashes, and pimples are also common for Pitta dosha.

Their lifelong vulnerability is to develop bleeding disorders, ulcers, and inflammatory conditions. Pitta individuals may struggle with negative emotions of jealousy and aggression, especially when experiencing an imbalance.

Pitta's attributes and manifestations

Attributes of Pitta	Physical and mental manifestations
Hot	Good appetite and digestion, warm body temperature, and intolerance to heat
Sharp	Good absorption and digestion, sharp memory, quick thinker, intelligent, brilliant, sharp teeth, and well-organized
Oily	Soft and oily skin, hair, and feces
Liquid	High thirst and sweat production, frequent urination, loose stools
Fluid	Charming, eloquent, and articulate well
Spreading	Acne, rashes, inflammation, well-known by others (popular)
Transforming	Great at implementing ideas, resourceful,

	analytical thought process
Intense	Intense emotions, passionate, strong feelings of anger and jealousy

Prevention of imbalance

Pitta **imbalance** can be prevented by avoiding aggravating factors, such as hot and humid weather, direct exposure to sunlight, salty and spicy foods, excessive work, smoking, and high consumption of caffeine and alcohol.

Skipping meals for a short time can make Pitta irritable and low on energy. It is recommended to eat shorter meals at regular intervals to avoid hunger. A high-intensity workout should be avoided during summer, especially in the afternoon. Proper hydration and cooling foods (like mint and cilantro) are remarkably helpful in maintaining balance. Pitta individuals can benefit immensely from regular meditation and calming yoga poses like the child pose, and the corpse pose.

For skin and hair, choose water-based hydration rather than oil-based creams. Light moisturizers like aloe vera, rose water, herbal hydrosols, coconut oil, jojoba oil, and argan oil are more suitable for Pitta skin.

Kapha-dominant mind-body type

Physical characteristics

As Kapha is the primary anabolic energy that builds muscles and tissues, people of this dosha are naturally blessed with well-built bones, a broad frame, and strong muscles. They are also well-endowed with beautiful facial features, prominent eyes, soft and smooth skin, long eyelashes, and thick and wavy hair. Their skin usually maintains an optimal amount of moisture and temperature. Kapha's pulse is noticeably slower than that of other doshas.

Kapha people tend to have the longest lifespan of all Prakriti types because of their slow metabolism. They encounter signs of aging quite later in life when compared to other dosha types. They have less food requirement but a fairly strong appetite, which makes them prone to weight gain.

Their ruling energy also gives them a strong immune system, healthful sleep, and well-functioning joints. Because of the heavy nature of Kapha, people of this dosha tend to sleep a lot.

Mental and emotional qualities

The nourishing nature of Kapha makes peaceful, empathetic, reliable, loving, sensitive, and grounded personalities. People close to them find their company very grounding and comfortable. Symbolic of the calm nature of the earth element, these individuals display a great degree of emotional stability even in turbulent times. They also display great control over their anger.

Kapha-dominant people are generally very goal-oriented and disciplined. They do not like unnecessary distractions and can find happiness in simple things. Their working style is slow-paced but very meticulous. Although they learn things relatively slower than Vata and Pitta, they possess excellent long-term memory.

Tendencies and vulnerabilities

Kapha individuals have a general inclination towards a sedentary lifestyle. They prefer less physical activity tasks, although they are naturally blessed with robust stamina. When coupled with a sedentary lifestyle and slow metabolism, a healthy appetite can make them prone to lifestyle disorders later in life.

With strong immunity and adaptability to weather changes, Kapha-dominant individuals do not experience too many health problems in their daily lives. However, they are vulnerable to mental health issues like loneliness, depression, low motivation, and heavy-heartedness. Their tendency to resist change can prevent them from seeking help.

Kapha people usually tend to hold water and weight. In case of imbalance, it can quickly escalate towards conditions like water retention and facial puffiness. Their lifelong vulnerability is obesity, diabetes, cardiovascular conditions, and depression.

Kapha's attributes and manifestations

Attributes of Kapha	Physical and mental manifestations
Liquid	Congestive disorders, edema, and mucus production
Hard	Firmness, solidity, compact and condensed tissues
Static	Preference for a sedentary lifestyle, fear of change, stubbornness
Viscous	Deeply attached to loved ones, values relationships
Slow	Slow speech and movement, steady appetite and thirst, sluggish digestion, and slow metabolism
Slimy	Excess salivation, prone to congestion
Cloudy	A foggy mind, especially in the morning upon awaking; often desires coffee for stimulation to start the day
Dense	Excellent bones with high mineral density, thick skin, hair, and nails
Soft	Smooth skin and hair, pleasant looking, prominent lips, well-endowed features, loving, caring, compassionate, and forgiving

Prevention of imbalance

Kapha imbalance can be prevented by avoiding sweets, raw and refrigerated foods, cold drinks, deep-fried and processed foods, refined carbs and fats, alcohol, and fat-rich dairy. Taking a short walk after meals can help improve digestion.

Kapha individuals benefit from well-spiced meals, which can help counter a sluggish metabolism. An ideal Kapha meal should be light and warm, prepared with dry cooking methods using a small amount of liquid.

For Kapha individuals, embracing an active lifestyle is vital for enjoying life to its fullest. They should develop an interest in sports, high-intensity training, strength training, dance, or other energizing practices. Stimulating yoga poses like the warrior pose and the cobra pose can help boost energy levels and bring balance.

Another important thing for Kapha is to establish a habit of rising early in the morning before sunrise. Practicing pranayama and sun salutation sequences can also help.

Kapha skin is naturally blessed with excellent moisture retention. They can benefit from light moisturizing oils like jojoba, sesame, argan, grapeseed, and aloe vera. Coconut oil triggers Kapha imbalances and should be avoided at nighttime.

Kapha individuals may face skin problems like blackheads and toxin buildup from time to time, which can be prevented by a proper exfoliation routine. Regular full-body detoxification can greatly improve the overall quality of life for this dosha.

Know your doshas!

This quiz has been designed for you to learn your unique mind-body type (Prakriti). It is important to understand that this quiz may not reflect your constitution accurately if the questions are not answered correctly. A constitutional assessment by an Ayurvedic physician or practitioner is the most accurate way of learning your dosha type. This quiz can, however, give you a fairly close idea of your dominant dosha.

Based on your lifetime tendencies, answer each question as accurately as possible. If there is more than one choice that looks relevant to you, choose the most prevalent in your state of optimal health and balance. Do not answer these questions based on circumstantial changes occurring in your life. This quiz is for assessing your personality type—not the current imbalance!

When all questions are answered, add up the scores in each column. The highest number is your dominant dosha. Now you may begin!

Doshic Quiz Form

Body structure	Body structure	Body structure
☐ Thin, bony frame, and difficulty gaining weight	☐ Medium frame and evenly distributed weight	☐ Large frame, heavy set frame, a tendency to gain weight easily
small bone structure	☐ medium bone structure	☐ heavy bone structure
Body Weight	**Body Weight**	**Body Weight**
☐ Gain weight more around the middle	☐ Gain or lose weight easily (weight is distributed evenly)	Gain weight more in the rear and thighs
Skin Type	**Skin Type**	**Skin Type**
☐ Dry, rough, and prone to cracking	☐ Soft, warm, and prone to freckles, acne, pimples, or moles	☐ Oily, thick, and prone to acne or blackheads
Hair	**Hair**	**Hair**
☐ Hair is dry, rough, scanty or over abundant	☐ Hair is light, soft or fine in hair texture, and prone to gray hair	☐ Hair is thick; may be slightly wavy, a little oily, dark brown, lustrous, and prone to dandruff
Sweat	**Sweat**	**Sweat**
☐ Sweat is scanty	☐ Sweat easily	☐ Sweat moderately and consistently
Eyes, size and color	**Eyes, size and color**	**Eyes, size and color**
☐ Eyes are small, darkeyes, sunken, and dry	☐ Eyes are medium size, light green, gray, blue, bright, sensitive to light, andare often red	☐ Eyes are large, blue or chocolate, moist, and prone to irritation or itchiness
Teeth shape and size	**Teeth shape and size**	**Teeth shape and size**
☐ Teeth are crooked, uneven, buck teeth, or may needbraces	☐ Teeth are even, or of medium size	☐ Large, even or shiny teeth
Gum	**Gum**	**Gum**
☐ Thin receding gum	☐ Gum bleeds easily	☐ Strong gum
Lips	**Lips**	**Lips**
☐ Small, dry lips	☐ Deep red lips	☐ Thick moist lips
Nails	**Nails**	**Nails**

☐ Hard, brittle rough nails; Irregular in shape and sizes	☐ Strong, soft nails, pink in color	☐ Nails are strong, large, symmetrical in size; may be pale in color
Pulse	Pulse	Pulse
☐ Pulse is fast or irregular	☐ Pulse is strong and full	☐ Pulse is steady, slow and rhythmic
Personality	Personality	Personality
☐ Talkative, restless, active	☐ Controlling; aggressive	☐ Calm, pleasant, quiet
Sex drive	Sex drive	Sex drive
☐ Sexual interest varies; active fantasy life is active	☐ Over-sexed and easily aroused	☐ Sex drive is steady, and slow to arousal
Sleep	Sleep	Sleep
☐ Sleep is light, or interrupted	☐ Sleep is deep, and tendency to oversleep	☐ Sleep is heavy, difficulty falling asleep, and tendency to snore
Appetite	Appetite	Appetite
☐ Irregular appetite, and can go long periods without food	☐ Good appetite, enjoy eating or always ready to eat	☐ Low or moderate appetite
Food preference	Food preference	Food preference
☐ Dry, raw, rich food, Irregular appetite and tendency to forget to eat	☐ Love proteins, caffeine, hot spicy foods, and tendency to eat at regular intervals	Love sweets, dairy, bread and pastry; have strong appetite and tendency to overeat or snack frequently
Thirst	Thirst	Thirst
☐ Less thirsty	☐ Frequently thirsty	☐ Less thirsty
Memory/Concentration	Memory/Concentration	Memory/Concentration
☐ Weak ability to concentration, good short-term memory, or forget quickly	☐ Good ability to concentrate, and good short and long-term memory	☐ Takes me time to learn, but good long-term memory and concentration
Organization discipline	Organization discipline	Organization discipline
☐ Disorganized, creative; dislike	☐ Very organized	☐ Work well with routine
☐ Unstable in making decisions or change my mind easily	☐ Make decision very quickly	☐ Take my time making decisions
Menstrual cycle	Menstrual cycle	Menstrual cycle

☐ Period may be painful and irregular	☐ Periods may be heavy and last longer, and may have loose stool	☐ Prone to water weight gain during my period, slight cramps, if any

Elimination	Elimination	Elimination
☐ Bowel movement can be Irregular, dry, hard or constipation day	☐ Loose bowel movement, or more than two a day	☐ Regular bowel movement; large soft stools
When Ill	When Ill	When Ill
☐ Sharp pain or nervous disorders	☐ Fever or inflammation	☐ Chest congestion, swelling, mucus, or water retention
Physical activity	Physical activity	Physical activity
☐ Very active and love to travel	☐ Love competitive activities	☐ Love leisure or activities that require less motion
Climate preference	Climate preference	Climate preference
☐ Warm, dry, and sunny	☐ Cool, damp, and cloudy	☐ Hot, humid, and tropical
Emotional and Mental	**Emotional and Mental**	**Emotional and Mental**
☐ Feelings and emotions are variable; or mood swings Prone to anxiety, worry, and fear	☐ Aggressive and give opinion even if it is not asked Prone to anger, frustration, and impatience	☐ Avoid giving opinion in difficult situations Prone to depression, lethargy, and sadness
	Anger, frustration, and impatience	Depression, lethargy, and sadness
Reaction stress	Reaction stress	Reaction stress
☐ Anxious, fearful, nervous, or jumpy	☐ Angry, short tempered; easily irritated	☐ Sensitive, passive, or sentimental
Energy level throughout the day	**Energy level throughout the day**	**Energy level throughout the day**
Moderate energy with peaks and valleys throughout the day	High energy and difficulty falling asleep at night	Low energy and difficulty waking up in the morning
Dreams	Dreams	Dreams
☐ Dreams involve flying; restless; nightmares	☐ Dreams are in color; fast; passion; conflicts	☐ Dreams are romantic and short

55

Total_____	Total_____	Total_____

Interpretation

If Vata has the highest score: You have a Vata constitution, and you tend to be creative, imaginative, and adaptable. However, you may also experience anxiety, nervousness, and difficulty focusing. Your physical characteristics may include a thin and light build, dry skin, and slow digestion.

If Pitta has the highest score: You have a Pitta constitution, you tend to be competitive, ambitious, and analytical. However, you may also experience anger, irritability, and impatience. Physical characteristics may include oily skin and hair, a strong appetite, and a moderate build.

If Kapha has the highest score: You have a Kapha constitution, which means you tend to be calm, easygoing, and loyal. However, you may also experience lethargy, weight gain, and difficulty letting go of things. Your physical characteristics may include a slow metabolism, oily and smooth skin, and a sturdy build.

Remember, this quiz is not intended to be a substitute for a constitutional assessment by an Ayurvedic physician or practitioner. Please consult a qualified healthcare professional if you have any concerns about your health or well-being.

Chapter 5

Nutrition and digestion

The Ayurvedic system of medicine, which originated in ancient India, emphasizes the role of food in achieving balance and promoting overall mental and physical wellness. According to Ayurveda, poor nutrition or the consumption of incompatible food is the root cause of all diseases. By eating in a way that best serves their needs, individuals can improve their health, extend their life, and prevent illnesses. In Ayurveda, food is regarded as medicine. However, if food is not adequately digested, it can become toxic and form a sticky substance that can accumulate in the tissues, ultimately leading to illnesses in the affected organs or systems over time.

The key to preventing disease and restoring health is consuming the right combination of foods to promote proper digestion. Ayurvedic nutrition is tailored to an individual's constitution, using a dietary regimen that considers the tastes, qualities, properties, and energetic effects of different foods on the body's doshas (Vata, Pitta, and Kapha), as well as their post-digestive effects on the tissues.

To balance the doshas with diet, choosing foods with opposite qualities is important. For example, those with excess Vata may benefit from warm, nourishing foods like soups and stews, while those with excess pitta may benefit from cooling foods like cucumber and mint. However, it's important to note that following a specific dietary regimen is not a one-size-fits-all approach, as every individual's body constitution is unique, and digestion is the foundation of good health.

Efficient digestion is critical for maintaining a healthy body, mind, and soul. If the digestive fire (agni) is too low, food takes longer to be absorbed, resulting in slow digestion. Conversely, if the digestive fire is too high, food burns too quickly, leading to digestive issues like acid reflux and heartburn. The proper function of agni should always be maintained within normal limits.

Several factors, including body constitution, time of day, season, location, age, and eating patterns, can affect an individual's metabolic function. According to Ayurveda, lunch should be the main meal of the day, consumed between 12 noon and 2 p.m. This is because the digestive fire is strongest during pitta time, making it easier to digest food. Eating late at night (after 8 p.m.) is not recommended, as it can cause toxins to accumulate in the body, leading to symptoms like fatigue and mucus in the throat.

Digestion: the key to perfect health

Digestion is considered the cornerstone of good health in Ayurvedic medicine. According to Ayurveda, perfect digestion is breaking down food into nutrients and the body's ability to assimilate and eliminate waste effectively. Digestive problems can lead to various health issues, including constipation, bloating, and nutrient deficiencies. Therefore, Ayurveda emphasizes the importance of optimal digestive health to achieve overall well-being.

The Ayurvedic concept of digestion is based on the idea of agni, which is often translated as "fire." Agni refers to the digestive fire responsible for breaking down food into its constituent parts. This fire is essential for digestion and is believed to be in the stomach and small intestine. According to Ayurveda, there are thirteen types of agni, each with a specific function and location in the body.

Digestion is treated in Ayurveda as not just a physical process, but also a mental and emotional one. In other words, the state of mind and emotions can affect the digestive process and vice versa. Stress, anxiety, and other negative emotions can impair digestion and lead to digestive disorders. Therefore, Ayurveda recommends a holistic approach to digestion that includes diet, lifestyle, and mental and emotional well-being.

Ayurvedic principles of digestion focus on balancing the three doshas: Vata, Pitta, and Kapha. Vata governs movement and is responsible for food movement through the digestive tract. Pitta governs metabolism and is responsible for the transformation of food into nutrients. Kapha governs structure and is responsible for the lubrication and nourishment of the digestive tract.

Therefore, Ayurveda recommends a diet appropriate for each person's unique constitution and digestive capacity. The diet should be tailored to balance the three doshas and promote optimal digestion. Foods that are easy to digest, such as cooked vegetables, soups, and stews, are recommended for those with weak digestion. Spices and herbs, such as ginger, cumin, and turmeric, are also used in Ayurvedic cooking to enhance digestion.

Ayurveda also recommends specific eating practices to support digestion. For example, eating in a calm and relaxed state of mind, chewing food thoroughly, and avoiding overeating can all improve digestion. Ayurveda also recommends avoiding cold or raw foods, which can dampen the digestive fire and impair digestion.

In addition to diet and eating practices, Ayurveda recommends lifestyle practices to support digestion. Regular exercise, stress management techniques, such as meditation and yoga, and adequate sleep are all important for optimal digestion. Ayurveda also recommends regular fasting or cleansing practices to support digestive health. Doing this helps individuals to achieve perfect digestive health and overall well-being.

The Digestive Fire

In traditional Ayurvedic medicine, the digestive fire is called "agni," which is considered essential to overall health and well-being. This digestive fire breaks down food, absorbs nutrients, and eliminates waste from the body. Ayurvedic practitioners believe a strong digestive fire is essential to maintaining optimal health, while a weak digestive fire can lead to various health issues.

The digestive fire is believed to be located in the stomach and small intestine and is responsible for converting food into a form the body can use. When the digestive fire is strong, it can break down food quickly and efficiently, extracting all the necessary nutrients while eliminating waste. This process is crucial for maintaining healthy body weight and preventing digestive issues such as bloating, gas, and constipation.

One of the secrets of good health, according to Ayurveda, is proper digestion. Your life essence, or Ojas, can flow freely in the circulatory channels when toxins, or ama, are minimal. Ojas is hindered when ama is high, which causes various health problems. This implies that life runs more easily when accumulated toxins do not burden your body and mind.

Low digestive "fire" (agni), which prevents your food from being adequately digested, the nutrients from being assimilated, and waste from being effectively expelled, leads to ama. This undigested food builds up in the stomach and intestines, where it can produce toxins like gas and bloating and cause candida overgrowth. It might eliminate the beneficial bacteria which would interfere with your digestion and metabolism. If we do not routinely remove toxins, we may become ill or, at the very least, experience a general feeling of tiredness.

Several factors can affect the strength of the digestive fire. One of the most important factors is the type of food that is eaten. In Ayurvedic medicine, foods are classified as "agni-enhancing" or "agni-reducing." Agni-enhancing foods are easy to digest and help increase the strength of the digestive fire. These include foods such as ginger, cumin, and fennel. Agni-reducing foods, on the other hand, are those that are difficult to digest and can weaken the digestive fire. These include processed foods, fried foods, and heavy meats.

Other factors that can affect digestive fire include stress, lack of sleep, and an imbalanced lifestyle. In Ayurveda, it is believed that stress and lack of sleep can weaken the digestive fire, as can an imbalanced lifestyle that includes too much activity or too little rest.

To maintain a strong digestive fire, Ayurvedic practitioners recommend eating a diet rich in agni-enhancing foods, practicing stress-reducing activities such as yoga and meditation, and getting plenty of rest. They also recommend avoiding agni-reducing foods and regularly eating throughout the day to keep the digestive fire burning strong.

Overall, the concept of digestive fire is an important one in Ayurvedic medicine. By paying attention to the strength of this vital function and taking steps to support it, individuals can improve their overall health and well-being.

How to maintain strong agni

Here are some tips for maintaining a strong agni:

- **Eat a balanced diet**: Eat foods that are easy to digest, such as cooked vegetables, soups, stews, and warm grains. Avoid heavy, oily, and processed foods that can slow down digestion.
- **Eat at regular intervals**: Eating at regular intervals helps to maintain a steady metabolic rate, which in turn helps to maintain a strong agni. Try to eat three meals a day at approximately the same time each day.
- **Sip warm water throughout the day**: Drinking warm water throughout the day helps to keep the digestive system hydrated and promotes proper digestion.
- **Exercise regularly**: Regular exercise helps to increase circulation, which improves digestion and promotes a strong agni.
- **Practice mindful eating**: Sit down and eat your meals in a calm and relaxed environment. This helps to reduce stress and promote proper digestion.

- **Reduce stress**: Stress can negatively impact digestion and weaken the agni. Try to manage stress through yoga, meditation, or deep breathing exercises.
- **Use herbs and spices**: Incorporating herbs and spices such as ginger, cumin, coriander, and fennel in your meals can help to promote a strong agni.

Remember, the strength of your agni is influenced by many factors, so it's important to take a holistic approach to maintaining good digestive health.

Six tastes: Elements, qualities, and doshas

Ayurveda teaches us that taste plays a critical role in maintaining the balance of our bodily doshas. Every type of food and medicinal herb has its own unique taste. When consumed in the right amounts, these tastes can work individually and together to help bring a sense of balance to our bodily systems.

Our tongue has taste buds organized into six groups, corresponding to the six tastes recognized by Ayurveda. These tastes are sweet, sour, salty, bitter, pungent, and astringent. Interestingly, these six basic tastes are derived from the five elements believed to form the basis of everything in the universe, including our body. The elements are space, air, fire, water, and earth.

Sweet taste is created by combining Earth and Water elements, sour taste by Earth and Fire, salty taste by Water and Fire, pungent or spicy taste by Fire and Air, bitter taste by Air and Space, and astringent taste by Air and Earth. Each taste uniquely affects our bodily systems, and their combination can synergistically affect our health and well-being.

When we consume food, the taste buds on our tongue perceive the taste and send a signal to the brain. From there, messages are sent out that directly influence our digestion and affect the doshas and all the body's cells, tissues, organs, and systems. This is why Ayurveda places great importance on taste and its effect on the body.

Understanding the properties of each taste and its effect on our body helps us make informed choices about what we eat and how we combine different tastes in our meals. For instance, a sweet taste is nourishing and grounding, while a sour taste can stimulate digestion and increase appetite. A salty taste can help to retain water in the body, while a bitter taste can aid in detoxification. A pungent or spicy taste can improve circulation and clear congestion, and an astringent taste can create a feeling of firmness and contraction in the body.

A well-balanced Ayurvedic diet would always have the six tastes (sad rasas). Excessive intake of one or the other rasas can tilt the equilibrium leading to a health problem. As an example, excessive intake of sweet-tasting foods can lead to obesity, pungent-tasting foods to acidity, etc. Therefore, incorporating a variety of tastes into our meals and using them in the right amounts allow us to balance our bodily systems and promote overall health and well-being. Ayurveda offers a comprehensive approach to understanding taste and its impact on the body, and this knowledge can help us make better choices about the food we eat and its effect on our health.

Tastes	Element	Action on Dosha	Qualities	Food Sources	Diseases
Sweet	Earth & Water	Vata ↓ Pitta ↓ Kapha ↑	Oily, cooling, and heavy	Fruits, légumes, grains, pasta, sugar, honey, molasses, dairy, and some cooked vegetables and meat	Obesity, excessive sleep, cough, fever, eye diseases, excessive mucus production
Sour	Earth & Fire	Vata ↓ Pitta ↑ Kapha ↑	Liquid, light, heating, and oily	Citrus or sour fruits, green grapes, kiwi, fermented foods such as pickles, tomatoes, vinegar, cheese, sour cream, and some salad dressings	Promotes thirst, sensitivity in teeth, blood disorders, burning sensation, generates heat in muscles, and suppurates wounds,

Salty	Water & Fire	Vata ↓ Pitta ↑ Kapha ↑	Heating, heavy, and oily	Natural salt, rock salt, black salt, sea salt, kelp, sea weeds, canned and processed foods, salt and water fish	Vitiates blood; causes skin diseases, internal bleeding, inflamma-tion, impotency, wrinkles in skin, gray hair, baldness
Bitter	Air & Ether	Vata ↑ Pitta ↓ Kapha ↓	Cool, light, and dry	Dark green leafy vegetables, olives, grapefruits, broccoli, sprouts, kale, and bitter melon, fenugreek leaves, turmeric...	Causes dryness of mouth and skin, reduces tissues, and obstructs channels, leads to emaciation and psychic disorders
Pungent	Fire & Air	Vata ↑ Pitta ↑ Kapha ↓	Light, drying, and heating	Chili, cayenne, long pepper and black	Causes burning sensation, impotency, giddiness,

				peppers, garlic, onion, cloves, ginger, radish, turnip, asafetida, and mustard	thirst, pain, tremors
Astrin-gent	Air & Earth	Vata ↑ Pitta ↓ Kapha ↓	Cooling, drying, and heavy	Unripe banana, green apples, grape skins, cranberries pomegra-nates, pears, cauliflower, artichoke, broccoli, Lentils, parsley turnip, rye, buckwheat quinoa, saffron, basil, turmeric and marjoram	Causes problems with normal speaking, flatulence, blackish discoloration, obstruct-tion of feces, urine, flatus, semen, spasms, convul-sions

Sweet Taste

The sweet taste is found in various foods, including rice, sugar, milk, wheat, dates, and maple syrup. When consumed in moderation, sweet foods can offer several health benefits. They are known to be oily, cooling, and heavy and can increase the vital essence of life.

In Ayurveda, an ancient system of medicine, the sweet taste is said to nourish and promote the growth of all seven Dhatus, which include plasma, blood, muscles, fat, bones, marrow and nerve tissue, and reproductive fluids. Doing so can give the body strength and longevity and promote healthy skin, hair, and a good voice. The sweet taste can also alleviate thirst and burning sensations and promote stability.

However, excessive consumption of sweet foods can lead to several health disorders. Sweet foods can heighten Kapha, which can cause colds, coughs, congestion, heaviness, loss of appetite, laziness, and obesity. They can also provoke lymphatic congestion, tumors, edema, diabetes, and fibrocystic changes in the breast.

It is important to note that not all sweet foods are created equal. Natural sweeteners like honey and jaggery, rich in vitamins and minerals, are healthier than refined sugar, which is high in calories and devoid of nutrients. It is also recommended to consume sweet foods in moderation and balance them with other tastes, such as sour, salty, bitter, and pungent, to maintain a healthy balance in the body.

Sour Taste

A sour taste is common in many foods, including citrus fruits, yogurt, vinegar, cheese, and fermented foods. These sour substances are liquid, light, heating, and oily. When taken moderately, they can be refreshing and delicious and offer various health benefits, such as boosting appetite and salivation, improving digestion, invigorating the body, nourishing the heart, and enhancing mental clarity.

Excessive consumption of sour taste, on the other hand, might have negative consequences on the body. Excessive thirst, hyperacidity, heartburn, acid indigestion, ulcers, and sensitive teeth are all possible side effects. The sour taste's fermenting activity may also be hazardous to the blood, resulting in skin disorders such as dermatitis, acne, eczema, boils, and psoriasis.

Furthermore, the hot nature of the sour taste can cause an acidic pH in the body, resulting in a burning sensation in the throat, chest, heart, bladder, and urethra. To avoid these negative consequences, it is critical to ingest sour flavor in proportion.

Salty Taste

Salt, a common seasoning used in almost all cuisines, comes in various forms, such as sea salt, rock salt, and kelp. It provides a distinctive salty taste that enhances the flavor of the food. However, excessive consumption of salt can lead to health issues.

In Ayurveda, salt is considered heating, heavy, and oily. When used in moderation, it can help relieve Vata dosha and increase Pitta and Kapha dosha. The water element in salt acts as a laxative, while the fire element helps to reduce spasms and pain in the colon. Salt also aids in digestion, absorption, and the elimination of waste.

Moderate salt consumption promotes growth and helps maintain water and electrolyte balance. It stimulates salivation and improves the overall taste of food. However, excessive salt consumption can aggravate Pitta and Kapha dosha. It can make the blood thick and viscous, causing hypertension and worsening skin conditions.

Overusing salt can also lead to various health problems, such as feeling hot, fainting, skin wrinkling, and baldness. It may also induce water retention and edema. Patchy hair loss, ulcers, bleeding disorders, skin eruptions, and hyperacidity are all possible consequences of overusing the salty taste.

Therefore, it is crucial to consume salt in moderation to avoid any adverse health effects. A balanced diet with adequate amounts of all the essential nutrients, including salt, can help maintain a healthy body and mind.

Bitter Taste

Bitter taste is commonly found in foods such as coffee, bitter melon, aloe vera, rhubarb, and different herbs such as yellow dock, fenugreek, turmeric root, dandelion root, and sandalwood. However, it is often the taste most lacking in the North American diet. Bitter taste is characterized as cool, light, and dry in nature. It increases Vata, while decreasing pitta and Kapha.

While bitter is not typically considered a delicious taste, it has several beneficial properties. For instance, it enhances the flavor of other tastes and is antitoxic, which helps to kill germs. Additionally, it is known to relieve itching, burning sensations, fainting, and obstinate skin disorders. A bitter taste is also known to reduce fever, promote firmness of the skin and muscles, and aid in digestion, particularly when consumed in small doses.

However, excessive consumption of bitter taste can cause a reduction in fat, bone marrow, urine, and feces, leading to extreme dryness and roughness, emaciation, and weariness. It can also deplete plasma, blood, muscles, fat, bone marrow, and semen, resulting in sexual debility. At times, excessive consumption of bitter taste can lead to dizziness and unconsciousness.

Pungent Taste

A pungent taste can be found in various foods, such as hot peppers like cayenne, chili, and black pepper, as well as onions, radishes, garlic, mustard, and ginger. In terms of quality, it has unique flavors of light, drying, and heating. Consuming pungent foods in moderation can have several health benefits, including improving digestion and absorption and cleansing the mouth. Additionally, it can stimulate nasal secretions and tearing of the eyes, helping to clear sinuses.

Moreover, a pungent taste is believed to aid circulation by breaking up clots, helping eliminate waste products, and killing germs and parasites. It can also bring clarity of perception. However, overuse of pungent foods in one's daily diet can have negative effects. It can kill sperm and ova, leading to sexual debility in both sexes. Overconsumption may also cause burning, choking, fainting, fatigue, and feelings of heat and thirst.

Pungency can aggravate Pitta, leading to diarrhea, heartburn, and nausea. Pungency is derived from both fire and air elements, and as a result, it can also aggravate Vata, leading to giddiness, tremors, insomnia, or pain in the leg muscles. Excessive use of pungent foods may result in peptic ulcers, asthma, colitis, and skin conditions. Therefore, consuming pungent foods in moderation is important to reap the benefits without experiencing negative effects.

Astringent Taste

An astringent taste is commonly found in unripe bananas, pomegranates, chickpeas, green beans, yellow split peas, okra, alfalfa sprouts, and various herbs such as goldenseal, turmeric, lotus seed, arjuna, and alum. This taste is characterized by a dry, choking sensation in the throat and has cooling, drying, and heavy properties.

When consumed in moderation, an astringent taste can calm the Pitta and Kapha doshas but may excite the Vata dosha. It is also known to promote the healing of ulcers and facilitate blood clotting.

However, excessive consumption of astringent foods may cause various side effects, including mouth dryness, speech difficulty, and constipation. It can also lead to abdominal distention, heart spasms, and circulatory stagnation. Prolonged overuse of astringent foods can result in a decrease in sex drive and sperm count. It can also lead to emaciation, convulsions, Bell's palsy, and neuromuscular Vata disorders.

Therefore, it is important to consume astringent foods in moderation and pay attention to any adverse effects that may occur. It is also important to maintain a balanced diet that includes a variety of tastes and to consult a healthcare professional if you have any concerns about your diet.

Food combining (incompatible foods)

Our food habits significantly impact our digestive health, and it is essential to be mindful of the food combinations we consume. In today's world, we are surrounded by various digestive aids and pills easily available in pharmacies and health food stores. However, many of these gastrointestinal problems are rooted in our food habits, particularly how we combine different foods. According to Ayurveda, improper food combinations can affect the normal functioning of our digestive fire, leading to an imbalance of the three doshas, namely Vata, Pitta, and Kapha.

Improper food combinations can result in various digestive issues such as indigestion, fermentation, putrefaction, and gas formation. These problems, when frequent or prolonged, can lead to serious health issues. For example, combining bananas with milk can diminish gastric fire or agni and change the intestinal flora, leading to the formation of toxins. This can cause sinus congestion, cold, cough, allergies, hives, and rash. Such disturbances generate ama, which is a toxic substance that is the root cause of most ailments.

To alleviate the ill effects of these combinations, you can use spices and herbs in your cooking. Spices such as ginger, cumin, coriander, and fennel can improve digestion and help to balance the doshas. A strong digestive fire can also be the most powerful means of dealing with these combinations. To stimulate digestion, you can chew a bit of fresh ginger sprinkled with salt and lime juice before meals.

Below is a chart of incompatible food to help individuals make informed dietary choices. It is worth noting that only some of the incompatible food combinations worth avoiding are listed in the chart. However, many other combinations can cause digestive issues, and it is best to consult an Ayurvedic expert to know more about them.

Incompatible Food Chart

Substances	Incompatible With
Beans	Cheese, curd, eggs, fish, fruits, meat, and milk
Black gram soup	Radish and jaggery
Chicken or meat	Dairy products
Curd	Cheese, eggs, fish, fruits, hot drinks, meat, milk and nightshades
Corn	Bananas, dates, and raisins
Eggs	Cheese, melons, beans, fish, fruits, milk, meat, yogurt, and curd.
Fruits	Milk and curd; must wait 30 minutes to 1 hour before consuming other food
Ghee	Kept in a bronze vessel for more than 10 days
Grains	Fruits and tapioca
Honey	With equal amount of ghee, should not be cooked or boiled
Jack fruit	Fish or seafood
Lemon	Cucumber, curd, milk and tomato
Melon	"Melon alone or leave it alone." Should not be eaten with other food.

Milk	Bananas, bread containing yeast, curd, yogurt, cherries, melons, sour fruits, fish, salt, and meat; drinking milk after eating radish or green leafy vegetables
Nightshades	Cucumber, melon, milk, and yogurt
Radishes	Bananas, milk, and raisins
Tapioca	Fruits, especially banana and mango, beans, raisins and jaggery
Wine	Curd and honey

Ayurvedic diet for each dosha

Ayurveda emphasizes the importance of maintaining a balanced and healthy diet to promote overall health and wellbeing. Its practitioners believe each person has a unique constitution, or dosha, which influences their physical, emotional, and mental characteristics. The three doshas are Vata, Pitta, and Kapha, and each requires a specific diet to maintain balance. Here is a brief overview of the Ayurvedic diet for each dosha:

Ayurvedic Diet for Vata Dosha

Vata is associated with air and space and is considered the most delicate of the three doshas. People with a predominant Vata dosha tend to be thin, with dry skin, brittle hair, and a tendency towards anxiety and worry. To balance Vata, the Ayurvedic diet should include warm, nourishing, and grounding foods such as:

Ayurvedic Diet for Vata

	Foods to Favor	Reduce or Avoid	Comments
Quality	Liquid: soup and stew	Light, cold, raw, and dehydrated foods	Warm milk, hot creamy cereals are good choices
Quantity	Eat 3-4 meals a day at regular times and intervals	Large portions	
Cooking Methods	Eat warm and creamy foods cooked in liquid	Baked and raw foods	
Pacify Tastes	Sweet, sour, and salty	Astringent, pungent and bitter	
Vegetables	Asparagus, avocado, beets carrots, cooked chilies (in very small quantities), cilantro, cucumber, garlic, green beans, green chilies, leeks,	Artichokes, beet greens, bell peppers, bitter melon, broccoli, brussels sprouts, cabbage, cauliflower, raw carrots, excess chili,	Steamed, stir-fried, stewed vegetables, or served with sauce to improve Vata digestive process. Raw

	mustard greens, okra, olives (black), cooked onion, parsnip, cooked peas, pumpkin, rutabaga, cooked spinach, summer squash, winter squash, sweet potatoes, watercress, zucchini	dandelion, eggplant, Jerusalem artichokes, green leafy vegetables, kohlrabi, lettuce, mushrooms, green olives, raw onions, raw peas, hot peppers, white potatoes, sprouts, tomatoes, turnips	vegetables and salads can be made more digestible and appetizing if marinated in olive oil and a pinch of salt or creamy dressing.
Fruits	Cooked apples, apricot, avocado, fully ripe banana, berries, cantaloupe, cherries, cantaloupe, coconut, dates, fresh figs, grapefruit, lemons, lime, grapefruit, grapes, kiwi,	Apple is astringent and can be drying for Vata. Unripe fruits because they are also astringent, dehydrated fruits, green banana, cranberries, dry dates, dried fruit in	All sweet ripe fruits are favorable; cooked apples with cinnamon and soaked dried fruits are acceptable.

	mangos, sweet melons, oranges, papaya, pineapple, peaches, plums, cooked or soaked prunes, raisins, tamarind, sour fruits, stewed fruits; all sweet and fully ripened fruits in general are good choices for Vata	general, pears, persimmons, pomegranate, dry prunes, dry raisins	
Grains	Amaranth, Durham flour, cooked oats, pancakes, multi grains, wheat, quinoa, white or basmati rice, seitan, sprouted wheat bread, wheat	Barley, buckwheat, corn, couscous, crackers, granola dry oats bran, millet and rye, muesli, pasta, rice cakes, spelt, tapioca, yeasted bread	Best to select whole grains to avoid food allergies and add crushed garlic, fennel, or cumin seeds to basmati rice to decrease gases

Dairy	Butter, buttermilk, organic whole milk if tolerated or goat milk, almond milk, cottage cheese, cream cheese and egg white, rice milk, oat milk, ghee, goat's milk, ice cream in moderation, sour cream in moderation, fresh yogurt,	Avoid dairy product in the case of lactose intolerance, frozen yogurt, powdered milk	If well tolerated, warm milk with spices such as cinnamon, anis star, cardamom, little sugar, or honey is very soothing for Vata and promotes good bowel movement
Meat	Chicken, turkey, and seafood; all in small quantity, duck, eggs, salmon,	Avoid red meat, difficult to digest	
Legumes	Chickpea, mung beans, pink or red lentils, tofu in moderation or small amounts, toor dal, urad dal	All, except as noted	Beans are excellent source of protein, but can be hard to digest; best to use split mung beans and red lentils

Oils	Avocado oil, castor oil, ghee, olive oil, safflower oil, sesame oil, and sunflower oil	Ghee if cholesterol is high, canola oil, corn oil, flax seed oil, soy oil	Mustard oil is good if used in modera-tion
Sweetener	Date sugar, raw honey, Raw brown sugar, agave syrup, maple syrup, molasses, sucanat, rice syrup, turbinado	Artificial sweeteners, white sugar, heated or cooked honey	
Nuts and Seeds	All are acceptable in small amounts; soaked are best.	Popcorn	
Herbs and Spices	Most spices are good for Vata if used in moderation: allspice, anise, asafetida, basil, bay leaf, *black pepper, caraway, cardamom, cilantro (coriander leaves), cinnamon,	Cayenne pepper, chili powder, fenugreek, horseradish, neem leaves	Use the following spices in small amounts: black, pepper, fenugreek parsley, saffron, and coriander seeds

	clove, cumin, fennel, fresh ginger, juniper berries, licorice root, mace, marjoram, mustard, nutmeg, oregano, sage, tarragon, and thyme		

Daily Routine and Self-Care: massage body with warm sesame oil, practice daily yoga, meditation, and spiritual healing; exercise should be passive or light.

Sleep Routine: follow a daily bedtime routine; go to sleep no later than 10 p.m.

Best Colors to Wear: red, yellow, orange and their shades

Aromatherapy: basil, clove, orange, geranium, and frankincense

Other: keep warm, calm and drink plenty of water daily, get plenty of rest and follow a regular schedule.

Ayurvedic Diet for Pitta Dosha

Pitta is associated with fire and is considered the most intense of the three doshas. People with a predominant Pitta dosha tend to be of medium build, with fair skin and a tendency towards anger and irritability. To balance Pitta, the Ayurvedic diet should include cooling, hydrating, and nourishing foods such as:

Ayurvedic Diet for Pitta

	Foods to Favor	Reduce or Avoid	Comments
Quality	Cool, lukewarm, and raw	Hot and over cooked foods	Pitta is the only dosha that digests raw foods well and easily
Quantity	Moderate proportion	Over eating	3-4 small-moderate portions daily
Method of Cooking	Moist heat and some baking		
Pacifying Tastes	Sweet, bitter, and astringent	Sour, salty and pungent	
Vegetables	Asparagus, broccoli, Brussels sprouts, cabbage, cucumber, cauliflower,	Beets, carrots, chili peppers, eggplant, garlic, onions, radishes, spinach, tomatoes	Vegetables can be combined with grains or mung beans and rice for a satisfying one-dish meal:

	celery, green beans, leafy greens, lettuce, mushrooms, okra, peas, potatoes, sprouts, zucchini		kitchari or vegetable biryani.
Fruit	Apples, avocado, *bananas, some berries, coconut, bananas, figs, sweet grapes, mango, melons, sweet oranges, pears, peaches, sweet pineapples, persimmon, sweet plums, pomegranate, prunes, raisins, and all sweet fruits are generally good for Pitta	Apricots, cherries, cranberries, grapefruit, limes, papaya, strawberries, and all sour fruits are to be avoided	Although banana is sweet, its post-digestive effect is sour, so eat in moderation.

Dairy	Buttermilk, ghee or unsalted butter, cottage cheese, yogurt, cow, or goat milk	Hard or aged cheese and sour cream	Milk, mango or mint lassi, young coconut juice and its meat
Herbs and Spices	Coriander, cumin, cinnamon, fennel, mint, and turmeric		Black pepper can be used in very small quantity
Legumes	Most legumes are ok		
Grains	Barley, cooked oats, basmati, brown and white rice, wheat	Buckwheat, corn, millet, dry oats and rye	Mung beans and rice, quinoa, or barley (kitchari) makes a delicious meal for Pitta.
Nuts	Coconut	Avoid all nuts	Nuts are very rich in oil, can aggravate Pitta
Oils	Coconut, olive, sunflower, and soy	Almond, corn, safflower, sesame	
Herbal teas and beverages	Alfalfa, chamomile, clove,	Ginger and other spiced drink	

comfrey, elderflower, fennel, jasmine, licorice, peppermint, organic fruit, and vegetable juices		

Daily Routine and Self-Care: massage body regularly with coconut oil, practice daily yoga, meditation, spiritual healing, and moderate exercises.

Sleep Routine: follow a daily bedtime routine to be in bed no later than 10 p.m.

Best Colors to Wear: blue, green, aqua and their shades

Aromatherapy: jasmine, sandalwood, rose and mint

Other: keep cool and calm; eat cooling, non-spicy food during summer and hot days; exercise during the coolest part of the day, such as early morning or after sunset, and avoid oily, salty, and deep-fried food.

Ayurvedic Diet for Kapha Dosha

Kapha is associated with earth and water and is considered the most stable of the three doshas. People with a predominant Kapha dosha tend to be of larger build, have oily skin, and have a tendency towards lethargy and depression. To balance Kapha, the Ayurvedic diet should include light, warming, and stimulating foods such as:

Ayurvedic Diet for Kapha

	Foods to Favor	Reduce or Avoid	Comments
Quality	Hot, warm, dry, light, spicy	Cold, raw, watery, and heavy	Foods for Kapha should be fully cooked
Quantity	Small-moderate portions	Over eating	Breakfast should be very light or a cup of tea with dry cereal is sufficient
Method of Cooking	Dry heat: roasted, baking or cooked in minimum amount of liquid	Foods cooked in too much liquid, oil	
Pacifying Tastes	Bitter, pungent, and astringent	Sour, salty and sweet	

Vegetables	Asparagus, bell peppers, broccoli, Brussels sprouts, cabbage, carrots, celery, eggplant, green beans, kale, leeks, lettuce, okra, onions, parsley, peas, spinach, and other leafy green vegetables	Avocado, beets, cauliflower, corn, cucumbers, mushroom, sweet potatoes, pumpkin, parsnip	Roots vegetables are very earthy; vegetables grown above the ground are better choice
Fruits	Apples, apricots, berries, cherries, cranberries, grapefruit, papaya, peaches, pears, pomegranate	Bananas, citrus, coconut, dates, figs, grapes, lemons, mangoes, oranges, plums, strawberries, and watermelon	
Dairy products	Goat milk, spiced buttermilk and skimmed milk in	Avoid all other dairy products, including cheese and yogurt	Dairy is too heavy and cooling for Kapha. Cumin or

	moderation and ghee in small quantity		ginger lassi can be taken occasionally; **see recipe on page**...
Herbs and spices	Ajwan, allspice, anise, asafetida, basil, bay leaf, black pepper, caraway, cardamom, cinnamon, cloves, coriander, cumin, dill, fenugreek, fennel, garlic, ginger, mace, marjoram, mint, mustard seeds, nutmeg, cooked onion, orange peel, oregano, paprika, poppy seeds (moderate amount), rosemary, sage, savory, spearmint,	Salt	Warming and stimulating herbs are the best choice for Kapha.

	star anise, tamarind, tarragon, thyme, vanilla, and wintergreen		
Legumes	Mung beans, red lentil, toor dhal, and soybean	Kidney beans, chickpeas, Soybeans	
Grains	Barley, corn, dry oats, millet, basmati rice, buckwheat, rye	Oats, other rice, wheat, pasta	Granolas, unsweetened dry cereals and puffed grains are good choice
Meat	Chicken, turkey, egg whites	Red meat and sweet and salt water fish	Shellfish are healing; stimulate Kapha
Nuts	Sunflower and pumpkin seeds	All other nuts and sesame seeds	
Oils	Corn, Mustard, sunflower	Almond, Avocado, Coconut, Olive, Sesame	Use oil in small amount
Herbal teas	Spiced herbal tea, fruits, or vegetable drinks	Cold or iced drinks, carbonated drinks, and alcohol	Ginger, cinnamon, and nutmeg tea to stimulate Kapha; black

			tea or coffee occasionally
Drinks	Warm drinks, fruit and vegetable juices, occasional tea, or coffee	Carbonated drinks, cold or iced drinks, alcohol	
Sweeteners	Raw honey	Avoid all other sweeteners	Use approximatel y one tablespoon per day; heated or cooked honey is very toxic to the body, so avoid that.

Guidelines for Balancing Kapha: Daily vigorous exercise (need encouragement to be receptive to useful change), periodic fasting is beneficial, varying daily routine, keeping active, avoiding daytime naps, and eating light meals; avoid cold meals and drinks, heavy, fatty, and acidic foods.

Daily Routine and Self-Care: Massage body with herbal powder; warm clove, eucalyptus, and juniper oil; exercise and prayer rituals.

Best Colors to Wear: red, orange, yellow and their shades.

Aromatherapy: basil, camphor or eucalyptus.

It is important to note that each person is unique, and their dosha may not fit perfectly into one of these categories. We recommend you consult with an Ayurvedic practitioner to determine your dosha and receive personalized dietary recommendations.

Identifying Ayurvedic energetics or qualities of foods (rasa, guna, vipak, virya, prabhav)

Ayurveda categorizes foods based on their energetics or qualities, referred to as "Panchamahabhutas" or five elements - earth, water, fire, air, and space. The five elements combine to form three doshas - Vata, Pitta, and Kapha- which govern the body's various physiological and psychological functions. The Ayurvedic energetics or qualities of foods can be described through the following parameters:

Rasa (Taste):

As reiterated earlier, Rasa refers to a particular food's taste. Ayurveda categorizes six tastes - sweet, sour, salty, pungent, bitter, and astringent. Each taste has a specific effect on the doshas and helps balance them. For example, a sweet and sour taste balances Vata, while a pungent and bitter taste balances Kapha.

Guna (Quality):

Guna refers to the physical and psychological qualities of a particular food. Ayurveda categorizes Gunas into ten pairs of opposite qualities: heavy-light, dull-sharp, oily-dry, cold-hot, etc. Each food has a dominant Guna, which affects the doshas differently. As an example, consuming heavy and oily foods can increase Kapha, while consuming light and dry foods can increase Vata.

Virya (Potency):

Virya refers to the heating or cooling effect of a particular food. Ayurveda categorizes virya into two types - hot and cold. The virya of foods affects the digestive fire or agni and influences the doshas. For example, consuming hot virya foods enhances Vata and Kapha, but aggravates Pitta because Pitta is hot. The hot virya promotes digestion, improves blood circulation, and increases body temperature. Whereas cold virya foods increase Vata and Kapha, but balances Pitta because of its cooling properties.

Vipak (Metabolism):

Vipak refers to the post-digestive effect of a particular food. Ayurveda categorizes vipak into three types - sweet, sour, and pungent. Vipak helps understand the digestive process and the effect of food on the doshas. As an example, sweet vipak foods balance Pitta and Kapha, while pungent vipak foods balance Vata.

Prabhav (Potency):

Prabhav refers to the unique or special effects of a particular food. Ayurveda considers prabhav the most important parameter as it defines the therapeutic effect of a particular food. An example of this is ginger, which is known for its ability to reduce inflammation and aid digestion.

Understanding foods' energetic qualities enables Ayurveda practitioners to recommend specific foods and dietary habits to balance the doshas and promote health and well-being. If someone has a Vata imbalance, which is characterized by dryness, anxiety, and insomnia, they would be recommended to eat warm, moist, and grounding foods like sweet potatoes, pumpkin, and cooked grains. Similarly, someone with a Kapha imbalance (characterized by sluggishness, weight gain, and congestion) might be advised to eat lighter, drier, and more pungent foods like bitter greens, ginger, and spices.

It's important to note that Ayurvedic dietary recommendations are highly individualized and depend on a person's unique constitution, health condition, and other factors. Therefore, it's best to consult a qualified Ayurvedic practitioner before making significant dietary changes.

Ayurvedic tips for eating well

According to Ayurveda, some foods might leave the body with harmful residue known as ama, which should be avoided. Frozen meals, leftovers that have been refrigerated for longer than 24 hours, processed foods, microwaved foods, and soups and sauces in cans with many ingredients should all be avoided. All of these foods contain less prana or life energy.

Here are a few fundamental Ayurvedic tips for eating well that you will find extremely beneficial:

- In the morning, start your day with hot water and a squeeze of a lemon or lime.
- Drink warm water or tea throughout the day.
- Eat three meals every day. Avoid eating snacks between meals. Following a meal, your body converts the food into energy and stores what is not immediately needed.

Your body can dig deep and draw on energy reserves to keep you running between meals. Even if you snack on carrots or apple slices all day, you are robbing your body of this necessary period of detoxification by not utilizing what is already present. If you frequently feel hungry between meals, you are probably not consuming enough meals that are high in nutrients. Occasionally, there might only be time for two meals due to timetable issues. That's all right, particularly for Kapha, who might function best with just two meals.

- Avoid combining fruit and other foods. Fruit should be consumed between 45 and an hour before any meal, particularly before breakfast. This isn't regarded as snacking. Your digestive juices will have plenty of time to assimilate the nutrients in the fruit before your main meal if you wait 45 mins to an hour.

- Avoid consuming cold fruits or drinks or raw salad vegetables. Avert ice.

- The body has a hard time processing raw food, which affects digestion. Cold food is the same way.

- Two open handfuls of food, or roughly two meals, should fill up around two-thirds of your stomach. (A person's stomach is typically larger than their hands.) In other words, eat until you are 80 percent full and save the remaining 20 percent for your body's internal "fires" to metabolize.

- Eat in moderation. After eating, you should feel energetic rather than bloated and drained. If you experience it, you either consumed too much food or combined it in a way that made it difficult to digest. It smothers the flame, like when you add too much wood to a fire. Consume just enough to keep your digestive system active! If the food you choose is nutrient-rich and simple to digest, two handfuls—similar to a big bowl—should be sufficient.

- Consume fewer grams of protein than are common in a Western diet. Eat little to no protein in the evening if any at all. You are probably eating more protein in the evening than you need unless you work the night shift, in which case your daily cycle is abnormal.
- Avoid mixing proteins. A buffet's array of options might be highly perplexing. Even if you stuff your face with many "good" things like beans, tofu, eggs, cottage cheese, and lean meats, your body is still under stress.
- Stick to one protein per meal as each one digests at a different rate.
- Consider lunch to be the most significant meal of the day. It should have the highest concentration of nutrients, such as protein and carbs. It is common to eat this lunch while working, but it is crucial that you pay attention to what you are eating. If possible, turn away from the computer and go outside to sit and eat.
- Make dinner the day's simplest meal to digest. If you must have protein with dinner, choose light proteins like fish, warm and prepared dishes, soups, and sautéed greens (which, strangely enough, have a relaxing effect). Eat dinner at least three hours before going to bed.
- Breakfast is significant, especially for Pitta and Vata, even though it isn't as crucial as the largest meal between 10 a.m. and 2 p.m. It should be warm, nourishing, and simple to digest for these types. A

simple serving of fruit or a light-grain porridge may be all that Kapha needs.

- Always eat when seated. Generally speaking, it's crucial to take the time to sit down and enjoy your meal if you want to be totally present. Enjoy your meal while sitting down and paying attention to what is on your plate. It doesn't count to eat while seated in your car.
- After meals, take a walk. After lunch and dinner, go for a quick walk to promote digestion.
- Try to sleep on your left side. It will facilitate digestion. Your major organs are supported, and your digestive fluids flow normally when you sleep on your left side.

Mahagunas

Mahagunas is a term used in Ayurveda to describe the three fundamental qualities that govern all aspects of the physical and mental universe. The Mahagunas are Sattva, Rajas, and Tamas, representing balance, activity, and inertia, respectively. These qualities are believed to be present in varying degrees in all living and non-living things and play a crucial role in determining an individual's physical and mental makeup. Understanding the Mahagunas and their interplay is essential in Ayurvedic diagnosis and treatment, as they help practitioners identify imbalances and create customized treatment plans that address the root cause of the issue. Through the use of Ayurvedic herbs, lifestyle modifications, and other therapies, practitioners aim to restore balance and harmony in the body, mind, and spirit, ultimately promoting optimal health and well-being.

Gunas as doshas of the mind

The mind is considered an essential component of human health and well-being in Ayurveda. According to Ayurveda, the mind comprises three Gunas: Sattva, Rajas, and Tamas. These Gunas are believed to play a significant role in determining the doshas of the mind and the personality traits associated with them.

Doshas are the fundamental energies in the body that govern the physical and mental aspects of human health. There are three primary doshas in Ayurveda, which are known as Vata, Pitta, and Kapha. Each dosha is associated with specific physical and mental characteristics, and imbalances in these doshas are believed to lead to various health problems.

Similarly, the Gunas of the mind are also associated with specific mental characteristics, and imbalances in these Gunas are believed to lead to psychological and emotional disorders. Let's take a closer look at each of these Gunas and how they relate to the doshas of the mind in Ayurveda.

Sattva Guna

Sattva Guna is the quality of purity, clarity, and balance. It is associated with the dosha of the mind called Vata, responsible for the nervous system's functions. In Ayurveda, it is associated with qualities of light, purity, and intelligence and provides mental clarity and a balanced perspective.

Sattva is derived from the Sanskrit word "sat," which means truth or existence. It represents a state of being in which the mind and body are in balance and harmony, allowing for the free flow of energy and information. This state of equilibrium enables us to access our inner intelligence, intuition, and wisdom.

When Sattva Guna is in balance within us, we are able to access our full potential and lead a life of purpose and fulfillment. We can maintain a clear and focused mind and subsequently make wise decisions that align with our true nature. This state of being also allows us to experience deep inner peace and contentment. A person with a predominant Sattva Guna tends to be calm, focused, and spiritually inclined.

In Ayurveda, several practices can help to cultivate Sattva, such as meditation, yoga, and a healthy lifestyle. These practices help calm the mind and body, reduce stress, and promote well-being. A healthy diet, regular exercise, and adequate sleep are also important for maintaining Sattva and promoting overall health.

However, when Sattva Guna is imbalanced, it can lead to anxiety, fear, and insecurity. A person with an imbalanced Sattva Guna may experience obsessive thoughts, depression, or mental fatigue.

Qualities of Sattva Guna

The qualities and attributes of Sattva Guna are many, and they manifest differently in each individual. Here are some of the most common attributes of Sattva Guna:

Clarity: People with a predominant Sattva Guna have a clear mind and a keen understanding of their nature and the world around them. They have a deep sense of purpose and can see the truth in all situations.

Calmness: Sattva Guna is associated with a calm and tranquil mind. People with a strong Sattva Guna are usually calm and collected in all situations. They are not easily disturbed or agitated and are able to maintain their composure even in difficult circumstances.

Compassion: Sattva Guna is also associated with compassion and empathy for others. People with a strong Sattva Guna can connect with others on a deep level and can understand and share their pain and suffering.

Contentment: Sattva Guna is characterized by contentment and satisfaction with one's life. People with a strong Sattva Guna can appreciate the simple things in life and are not driven by materialistic desires.

Discipline: Sattva Guna is also associated with discipline and self-control. People with a strong Sattva Guna can control their thoughts and emotions and can follow a disciplined and structured lifestyle.

Joy: Sattva Guna is also associated with joy and happiness. People with a strong Sattva Guna are able to find happiness in small things and can maintain a positive attitude toward life.

How Sattva Guna Manifests in You

Sattva Guna manifests in people in the following ways:

Clarity of Mind: People with dominant Sattva Guna have a clear and focused mind. They are able to think clearly and make decisions with ease.

Emotional Balance: They are emotionally balanced and have a positive outlook on life. They are not easily swayed by negative emotions such as anger, fear, or jealousy.

Compassion and Empathy: Sattvic people are compassionate and empathetic towards others. They can understand and connect with people on a deeper level.

Love for Nature: They have a deep appreciation and love for nature. They often spend time in nature, which helps to calm their mind and restore their inner balance.

Health and Well-being: People with dominant Sattva Guna tend to have good physical and emotional well-being. They have a healthy lifestyle, eat a balanced diet, and exercise regularly.

Spiritual Growth: They strongly desire spiritual growth and seek to connect with their inner self. They are often drawn toward spiritual practices such as spiritual healing, meditation, yoga, tai chi, qigong, or prayer.

Creativity: Sattvic people are often creative and express themselves through art, music, or other forms of creative expression. They are able to tap into their inner creativity and express it in a positive way.

Selflessness: They are selfless and always willing to help others. They derive joy from serving others and positively impacting the world.

In summary, people with a dominant Sattva Guna exhibit a balanced, positive, and harmonious nature. They lead a fulfilling life and positively impact the world around them.

Rajas Guna

Rajas Guna is the quality of activity, passion, and desire. It is associated with the dosha of the mind called Pitta, which is responsible for the metabolic processes in the body. This Guna is associated with qualities of motion, energy, and passion, and it is responsible for providing us with the ability to take action, experience emotions, and engage with the world around us.

Rajas is derived from the Sanskrit word "raj," which means to shine or glow. It represents a state of being with movement and activity, allowing for expressing our desires and passions. This energy is what drives us to pursue our goals and engage with the world in a dynamic and creative way.

When we cultivate Rajas within ourselves, we are able to take action and make things happen. We are able to experience the full range of human emotions, including love, joy, anger, and sadness. This energy also enables us to engage with the world through our senses, experiencing the beauty and wonder of the world around us. When Rajas Guna is balanced, it is associated with qualities such as motivation, creativity, and ambition. A person with a predominant Rajas Guna tends to be energetic, dynamic, and goal-oriented.

However, when Rajas Guna is imbalanced, it can lead to anger, aggression, restlessness, and an inability to focus. When overwhelmed by this energy, we may find ourselves constantly chasing after new experiences and unable to find inner peace and contentment. A person with an imbalanced Rajas Guna may experience irritability, impulsiveness, or hyperactivity.

Practices such as spiritual healing, meditation, yoga, tai chi, qigong, and mindfulness, can help to balance Rajas. These practices help to calm the mind and reduce the excess energy of Rajas, promoting a sense of inner peace and balance. A healthy diet, regular exercise, and adequate rest are important for maintaining balance and promoting overall health.

Qualities of Rajas Guna

The qualities and attributes of Rajas Guna are many, and they manifest differently in each individual. Here are some of the most common attributes of Rajas Guna:

Restlessness: People with a predominant Rajas Guna tend to be restless and agitated. They are always on the move and find it difficult to sit still or relax.

Ambition: Rajas Guna is associated with a strong desire for success and recognition. People with a strong Rajas Guna are usually ambitious and driven to succeed in their goals.

Passion: Rajas Guna is characterized by a strong passion for life. People with a strong Rajas Guna are enthusiastic and energetic and often throw themselves wholeheartedly into their work and relationships.

Impulsiveness: People with a strong Rajas Guna tend to be impulsive and act without thinking. They often take risks and are not afraid to challenge themselves.

Attachment: Rajas Guna is also associated with a strong attachment to material possessions, relationships, and achievements. People with a strong Rajas Guna tend to be possessive and can be jealous of others they perceive as threats to their success.

Aggression: People with a strong Rajas Guna can sometimes be aggressive or confrontational in their behavior. They may become angry or frustrated easily and can lash out at others.

How Rajas Guna Manifests in You

Rajas Guna manifests in people in various ways, including:

Hyperactivity: People with dominant Rajas Guna tend to be hyperactive and constantly on the move. They find it difficult to sit still and often feel the need to be engaged in some activity.

Competitive nature: Individuals with Rajas Guna strongly desire to compete and win. They are often driven by ambition and strive to be the best in their chosen field.

Impulsivity: People with Rajas Guna tend to be impulsive and act without much thought. They may make hasty decisions and regret them later.

Aggression: Individuals with Rajas Guna can be aggressive and confrontational. They may get into arguments and fights easily.

Inability to relax: People with dominant Rajas Guna find relaxing difficult and may have trouble sleeping. They are always on the go and feel restless when not doing anything.

Restlessness: Rajas Guna individuals may experience restlessness and a sense of unease. They may feel that something is missing in their lives and constantly seek new experiences and challenges.

Workaholism: People with Rajas Guna may become workaholics and put all their energy into their work. They may neglect other aspects of their lives, such as family and relationships.

Overindulgence: Individuals with dominant Rajas Guna may indulge in excessive behaviors such as overeating, overspending, or indulging in addictive substances.

To balance the effects of Rajas Guna, individuals are advised to adopt a more Sattvic lifestyle that includes practices such as meditation, yoga, and self-reflection. They can also benefit from a balanced diet, adequate rest, and engaging in creative and calming activities.

Tamas Guna

Tamas Guna is the quality of inertia, darkness, and ignorance. It is associated with the dosha of the mind called Kapha, which is responsible for the body's structural integrity. In Ayurveda, Tamas Guna allows us to rest, recuperate, and experience a deep sense of peace. A person with a predominant Tamas Guna tends to be peaceful, grounded, and dependable.

Tamas is derived from the Sanskrit word "Tamah," which means darkness or ignorance. It represents a state of being in which there is a lack of movement or activity, allowing for the rest and rejuvenation of the mind and body. This energy enables us to experience deep sleep and restore our energy levels.

However, an imbalanced Tamas Guna can lead to feelings of lethargy, apathy, and confusion. When overwhelmed by this energy, we may find ourselves unable to take action or make decisions and struggle to find motivation or direction in our lives.

In Ayurveda, practices such as meditation, yoga, and regular exercise, help to balance Tamas. These practices help to increase our energy levels and reduce the excess energy of Tamas, promoting a sense of vitality and clarity. A healthy diet, regular sleep, and a balanced lifestyle are also important for maintaining balance and promoting overall health.

Qualities of Tamas Guna

The qualities and attributes of Tamas Guna are many, and they manifest differently in each individual. Here are some of the most common attributes of Tamas Guna:

Laziness: People with a predominant Tamas Guna tend to be lazy and lethargic. They lack motivation and find it difficult to get things done.

Apathy: Tamas Guna is associated with a lack of interest in life. People with a strong Tamas Guna may be disinterested in relationships, work, or other aspects of their life.

Delusion: Tamas Guna is characterized by a state of delusion or confusion. People with strong Tamas Guna may be unable to see the truth or be easily deceived by others.

Inertia: Tamas Guna is associated with a state of inertia or stagnation. People with a strong Tamas Guna may find it difficult to change their lives or move forward.

Ignorance: Tamas Guna is also associated with a lack of knowledge or understanding. People with strong Tamas Guna may be ignorant of important facts or resist learning new things.

Attachment: Tamas Guna is characterized by a strong attachment to comfort and familiarity. People with strong Tamas Guna may resist change and prefer to stay in their comfort zone rather than take risks.

How Tamas Guna Manifests in You

Tamas Guna manifests in people in various ways, including:

Physical symptoms: Tamas Guna can manifest in physical symptoms such as fatigue, sluggishness, and a lack of energy.

Emotional symptoms: People with Tamas Guna may experience emotional symptoms such as apathy, lack of motivation, and a general feeling of heaviness or depression.

Poor decision-making: Tamas Guna can lead to poor decision-making and clarity, as the mind becomes clouded with lethargy and confusion.

Indulgence in unhealthy habits: People with Tamas Guna may be prone to indulging in unhealthy habits such as overeating, oversleeping, and excessive consumption of alcohol or drugs.

Resistance to change: Tamas Guna can make people resistant to change, as they may feel comfortable in their current state of inertia and be unwilling to take action to improve their situation.

In conclusion, the Gunas of the mind in Ayurveda is believed to play a crucial role in determining the doshas of the mind and the personality traits associated with them. A balanced state of the Gunas is essential for maintaining mental and emotional well-being; imbalances in the Gunas can lead to various mental health problems. Understanding the Gunas and their relationship with the mind's doshas can help individuals identify their mental constitution and make appropriate lifestyle choices to maintain balance and harmony.

Sattvic, Rajastic and Tamasic Food

	Sattvic foods	Rajasic foods	Tamasic Foods
Nature	Light and easy to digest, promote spiritual growth: qualities of peace, contentment, mercy, compassion	Promotes anger, hatred, irritability, stimulation, and agitation the mind	Induces sleep and promotes depression
Qualities of Foods	Fresh, juicy, unctuous, nourishing, sweet and tasty foods rich in prana (life force)	Sour, bitter, salty, pungent, dry, hot	Dehydrated, heavy, stale, old and processed foods
Examples	Rice, milk, fresh locally grown/organic fruits and vegetables, ghee, sprouted beans, grains, nuts, herbs and spices, compatible foods, and combinations	Deep fried food, red meat, high protein food, garlic, onion, chili pepper, coffee, and other stimulants	Beef, onion, leftover foods, canned, processed food, aged cheese, and egg yolk
Action	Spiritual	Stimulate	Create

	Essence, brings clarity and consciousness	desire and uncontrollable greed and attachment	pessimism, dullness, heaviness, drowsiness

Detoxification of the mind

Detoxification of the mind is a process of removing negative or toxic thoughts, emotions, and behaviors from one's mental state. In Ayurveda, the traditional Indian system of medicine, the three Mahagunas (Sattva, Rajas, and Tamas) are believed to play a crucial role in detoxifying the mind.

Sattva, Rajas, and Tamas are the three primary qualities or Gunas that exist in everything in the universe, including our mind and body. Sattva is associated with purity, clarity, and peace, Rajas with activity, passion, and restlessness, and Tamas with inertia, darkness, and ignorance.

To detoxify the mind through these three Mahagunas, Ayurveda suggests the following:

Sattva: To begin detoxifying the mind, it is essential to increase the Sattva Guna. Sattva Guna refers to the quality of purity and positivity that exists within us. We can experience a clearer mind and greater inner peace when we increase this quality.

One of the most effective ways to enhance the Sattva Guna is through meditation. By taking the time to sit in silence and focus our attention on our breath, we can calm our minds and increase our sense of inner tranquility.

Practicing yoga is another powerful method for cultivating Sattva Guna. Through various physical postures and breathing techniques, we can improve our physical health, release tension and stress, and promote mental clarity and focus.

Pranayama, or breathing exercises, can also enhance the Sattva Guna. By controlling our breath and directing our focus inward, we can increase our energy levels, boost our mental clarity, and release negative emotions.

In addition to these practices, paying attention to our diet is essential. Consuming a Sattvic diet consisting of fresh, natural, and pure foods can help us detoxify our bodies and minds. Sattvic foods include fruits, vegetables, grains, nuts, and other whole foods that are minimally processed and free from additives and preservatives.

By combining these practices and incorporating Sattvic foods into our diets, we can create a foundation of purity and positivity within ourselves, which can help us to detoxify our minds and live a more fulfilling and balanced life.

Rajas: After increasing the Sattva Guna, the second step in detoxifying the mind is to reduce the Rajas Guna. Rajas Guna refers to the quality of passion, activity, and restlessness within us. When this quality is excessive, it can lead to agitation, stress, and anxiety.

To reduce the Rajas Guna, it is essential to avoid stimulants such as caffeine and alcohol. These substances can increase our heart rate and blood pressure, which can lead to feelings of restlessness and anxiety. Instead, opt for herbal teas or other calming beverages.

It is also important to reduce the time spent on overly stimulating activities. For example, limit your screen time, including time spent on electronic devices such as computers, smartphones, and tablets. These activities can overstimulate our minds and make it difficult to relax and unwind.

Another way to reduce the Rajas Guna is to engage in activities that promote relaxation and calmness, such as taking a warm bath, practicing gentle yoga, or stretching, or spending time in nature. These activities can help to slow down our thoughts and promote a sense of inner peace.

Regular exercise can also be an effective way to reduce the Rajas Guna. Engaging in activities such as walking, jogging, or swimming can help to release pent-up energy and promote a sense of calm and relaxation.

Finally, it is essential to prioritize relaxation in our daily lives. This may involve setting aside time for meditation, taking a nap, or simply taking a break from our busy schedules to enjoy some quiet time alone.

By reducing the Rajas Guna and promoting a sense of calm and relaxation within us, we can cultivate greater inner peace and balance, which can help us to detoxify our minds and live a more fulfilling life.

Tamas: The third and final step in detoxifying the mind is eliminating the Tamas Guna. Tamas Guna refers to the quality of darkness, inertia, and lethargy within us. When this quality is excessive, it can lead to feelings of laziness, apathy, and depression.

To eliminate the Tamas Guna, avoiding heavy, oily, and processed foods is essential. These foods can make us feel sluggish and lethargic, making it difficult to maintain a sense of vitality and energy. Instead, opt for lighter, more nourishing foods such as fresh fruits and vegetables, whole grains, and lean proteins.

Getting regular exercise is another effective way to eliminate the Tamas Guna. Exercise can help to increase our energy levels and reduce feelings of inertia and laziness. Even a short walk or gentle yoga practice can promote a sense of vitality and well-being.

In addition to diet and exercise, it is important to prioritize rest and sleep in our daily lives. Lack of sleep and rest can contribute to feelings of lethargy and depression, so get enough rest and allow time for relaxation in your daily routine.

Meditation and other mindfulness practices can also be beneficial in eliminating Tamas Guna. These practices can help us become more aware of our thoughts and emotions and promote a sense of clarity and focus that can help overcome feelings of lethargy and apathy.

Finally, it is important to cultivate a positive mindset and surround ourselves with positive influences. This may involve spending time with supportive friends and family, engaging in activities that bring us joy and fulfillment, and practicing gratitude and self-care regularly.

By eliminating the Tamas Guna and promoting a sense of vitality and energy within us, we can cultivate greater inner strength and resilience, which can help us to overcome obstacles and achieve our goals in life. Focusing on these three Mahagunas and incorporating these practices into one's daily routine makes it possible to detoxify the mind and experience greater clarity, peace, and well-being.

Cultivating sattvic qualities

According to Ayurveda, one of the keys to maintaining health is the proper elimination of toxins from the body. In addition to specific dietary and lifestyle practices, Ayurveda recommends cultivating sattvic qualities such as compassion, forgiveness, and gratitude to enhance the detoxification process further.

Sattva is one of the three Gunas or qualities of nature, according to Ayurveda. It represents purity, harmony, and balance. By cultivating sattvic qualities, we can promote balance and harmony in our physical, emotional, and spiritual selves, leading to greater well-being.

Compassion is a virtuous trait that involves having empathy and understanding towards both you and others. When we develop compassion, we establish a stronger connection with the world, which can bring a greater sense of peace and harmony within us.

Forgiveness is another sattvic quality that involves letting go of resentment, anger, and grudges towards the self and others. By practicing forgiveness, we release negative emotions and thoughts that can create blockages in our energy and inhibit the body's natural ability to heal.

Gratitude is a third sattvic quality that involves acknowledging and appreciating the good things in our lives, no matter how small. The cultivation of gratitude allows us to shift our focus from what we lack to what we have, leading to greater contentment and peace of mind.

To achieve optimal health and vitality, it is essential to cultivate sattvic qualities such as empathy, forgiveness, and gratitude.

Creating a nurturing and uplifting environment promotes detoxification and fosters inner harmony, leading to a healthier, more energized life. Let us prioritize these qualities and work towards a better world and a better self.

Importance of mindful living

Ayurveda is based on achieving balance and harmony in all aspects of life. One of the key concepts in Ayurveda is that of the Mahagunas or the three great qualities that exist in everything in the universe, including our bodies and minds. These qualities are Sattva, Rajas, and Tamas, which are believed to influence our physical, emotional, and spiritual well-being.

Sattva, the quality of purity and clarity, is associated with feelings of peace, contentment, and happiness. Rajas, the quality of activity and restlessness, is associated with energy, passion, and drive. Tamas, the quality of inertia and darkness, is associated with lethargy, laziness, and depression. According to Ayurveda, we experience good health and well-being when these qualities are balanced. However, excess of these qualities can lead to physical or emotional imbalances and health issues.

Mindful living is an important component of Ayurveda because it helps us to stay connected to our true selves and to maintain balance in our lives. When we live mindfully, we become more aware of our thoughts, feelings, and actions and make choices supporting our physical, emotional, and spiritual health. This awareness allows us to recognize when we are experiencing an excess of Rajas or Tamas and take steps to bring ourselves back into balance.

For example, when experiencing excess Rajas, we may feel restless, anxious, or overwhelmed. By practicing mindfulness, we can become aware of these feelings and take steps to calm our minds and bodies. This may involve taking a break from a stressful situation, practicing deep breathing or meditation, or engaging in a relaxing activity like yoga or Tai Chi.

Similarly, when experiencing an excess of Tamas, we may feel sluggish, lethargic, or unmotivated. Living mindfully helps us recognize when we are feeling this way and take steps to increase our energy and motivation. This may involve regular exercise, eating a healthy and balanced diet, or engaging in activities that bring us joy and inspiration.

Living in a state of Sattva, or purity and clarity, is the ultimate goal of Ayurveda. When we cultivate this quality, we are able to experience a sense of peace, contentment, and well-being. Mindful living is essential to achieving this state, as it allows us to become more aware of ourselves and our surroundings and make choices that support our physical, emotional, and spiritual health. In addition to mindfulness practices, Ayurveda offers a range of natural remedies and treatments to support the body's natural healing process, including herbal medicines, massage, and yoga therapy.

Therefore, mindful living enables people to manage stress, cope with serious illness better, and reduce anxiety and sadness. Its practice leads to improved relaxation abilities, increased zest for life, and higher self-esteem.

How to Lead a Balanced Life

How seasons and time of the day influence health

According to Ayurveda, seasons and the time of the day can significantly impact our health. Ayurveda recognizes three primary doshas, or bodily humor, that govern the body's functions: Vata, Pitta, and Kapha. Each dosha is associated with specific seasons and times of the day, and understanding these connections can help us maintain balance and promote good health.

Seasonal Influence:

Vata Season: In Ayurveda, Vata is one of the three doshas or energies that govern the body and mind. It is associated with movement, creativity, and vitality. However, when Vata is imbalanced, it can cause physical and mental symptoms such as dry skin, constipation, anxiety, and restlessness.

During the Vata season, usually between the autumn and early winter months (September-December), the dry and cold weather can aggravate Vata, leading to further imbalances. Therefore, following a Vata-pacifying diet and lifestyle is recommended to maintain balance and promote overall health and well-being.

A Vata-pacifying diet includes warm and nourishing foods such as cooked grains, soups, stews, and root vegetables. Incorporating healthy fats such as ghee or coconut oil into your diet and warming spices like ginger, cinnamon, and cumin is also beneficial.

Engaging in gentle exercises, such as yoga or walking, can also help balance Vata during the season. It is important to avoid overexertion, as this can further aggravate Vata.

Other practices that can help balance Vata during the season include regular self-massage with warm oil, practicing mindfulness and relaxation techniques, and maintaining a regular sleep schedule.

Pitta Season: In Ayurveda, Pitta is associated with fire, transformation, and digestion. However, imbalanced Pitta can cause physical and mental symptoms such as inflammation, heartburn, irritability, and anger.

During the Pitta season, usually between the summer months (June-August), the hot and humid weather can aggravate Pitta, leading to further imbalances. Therefore, following a Pitta-pacifying diet and lifestyle is recommended to maintain balance and promote overall health and well-being.

A Pitta-pacifying diet includes cooling and hydrating foods such as cucumbers, watermelon, coconut water, and leafy greens. It is also beneficial to incorporate sweet, bitter, and astringent tastes into your diet while avoiding spicy, sour, and salty foods.

Calming activities such as swimming, spending time in nature, and practicing meditation can also help balance Pitta during the season. Avoiding overexertion and exposure to direct sunlight is important, as this can further aggravate Pitta.

Other practices that can help balance Pitta during the season include drinking plenty of water, wearing loose and light-colored clothing, and avoiding the consumption of alcohol and caffeine consumption. Maintaining a regular sleep schedule and practicing stress-reducing techniques is also important.

Kapha Season: Kapha is associated with stability, grounding, and nourishment. However, when Kapha is imbalanced, it can cause physical and mental symptoms such as lethargy, weight gain, congestion, and depression.

During the Kapha season, usually between the late winter and early spring months (January-April), the cold and damp weather can heighten Kapha, leading to further imbalances. Therefore, following a Kapha-pacifying diet and lifestyle is recommended to maintain balance and promote overall health and well-being.

A Kapha-pacifying diet includes light and warming foods such as ginger tea, spicy soups, and light grains like quinoa and millet. Incorporating pungent, bitter, and astringent tastes into your diet while avoiding sweet, sour, and salty foods is also beneficial.

Vigorous exercise like running or biking can also help balance Kapha during the season. Avoiding sedentary activities and getting plenty of fresh air and sunlight is important.

To balance Kapha during the season, try dry brushing, yoga, and avoiding too much sleep. Stick to a routine and do activities that engage your mind and body, like reading or learning something new.

Time of Day Influence:

Vata Time: The hours between 2-6 am and pm are considered the Vata time, as these times of day are characterized by the qualities of Vata - movement, change, and creativity. To balance Vata during these hours, engaging in calming activities that promote relaxation and grounding is recommended.

To effectively balance Vata during specific times of the day, it is imperative to engage in practices such as meditation, yoga, and breathing exercises. These activities not only promote mindfulness but also have the ability to reduce stress and calm the mind and body. It is highly recommended to avoid any activities that may stimulate the mind and body, such as using electronic devices, watching TV, or engaging in intense physical activity.

Other practices that can help balance Vata during these hours include taking a warm bath, practicing self-massage with warm oil, and drinking warm tea or milk before bed to promote relaxation and restful sleep. Maintaining a regular sleep schedule and creating a calm and peaceful environment in the bedroom is also important.

Pitta Time: The hours between 10 am-2 pm and 10 pm-2 am are considered Pitta time, as these times of day are characterized by the qualities of Pitta - digestion, metabolism, and focus. To balance Pitta during these hours, engaging in practices that support healthy digestion and promote relaxation is recommended.

Eating light and cooling foods like salads and fresh fruits can help balance Pitta during the day. It is important to avoid heavy, oily, and spicy foods that can aggravate Pitta and lead to digestive issues. Drinking plenty of water and herbal teas can also help support healthy digestion.

Kapha Time: In Ayurvedic medicine, the hours between 6-10 am and pm are considered the Kapha time, as Kapha dosha is dominant during this time. Kapha is one of the three doshas in Ayurveda, representing stability, strength, and growth. However, an excess of Kapha can lead to sluggishness, lethargy, and weight gain.

To balance Kapha during these hours, engaging in invigorating activities such as exercise is recommended. Exercise can help to stimulate metabolism, increase circulation, and promote energy and vitality. Some suitable exercises during Kapha time include brisk walking, running, or cycling.

Additionally, it is recommended to eat warming foods such as oatmeal or eggs to balance Kapha. These foods help to stimulate the digestive fire, improve metabolism, and provide sustained energy throughout the day. Other warming foods consumed during Kapha time include ginger tea, hot soups, and spicy dishes.

Individuals can maintain balance in their Kapha dosha by engaging in invigorating activities and consuming warming foods during Kapha time, promoting energy, vitality, and overall well-being.

In conclusion, Ayurveda suggests that understanding the connection between seasons and the time of day can help us maintain balance and promote good health. Adjusting our lifestyle according to these guidelines can improve our overall well-being and avoid imbalances that may lead to disease.

Preventing imbalance through the right lifestyle (living in harmony with nature)

Ayurveda is a holistic approach to health that prevents imbalance in the body, mind, and spirit through lifestyle choices that promote harmony with nature. According to Ayurvedic principles, imbalances in the body can lead to disease and illness, and the best way to prevent these imbalances is to live in harmony with nature.

Living in harmony with nature means making choices that support your body's natural rhythms and needs. Ayurveda teaches that each person has a unique constitution or "dosha," which comprises of: Vata, Pitta, and Kapha. These doshas govern different aspects of the body, and an imbalance in any of them can lead to illness or disease.

Here are some Ayurvedic lifestyle practices that can help prevent imbalance and promote harmony with nature:

Eat a balanced diet: Ayurveda emphasizes the importance of a balanced diet tailored to an individual's dosha or unique constitution. Each dosha has its own unique set of characteristics and is associated with certain physical and mental qualities.

To eat a balanced diet according to your dosha, choose foods that help balance and harmonize your specific dosha. For example, someone with a Vata constitution, which is associated with coldness, dryness, and instability, may benefit from warm, nourishing foods that are easy to digest, such as soups and stews made with root vegetables, grains and warming spices like ginger and cinnamon. They should also eat naturally sweet, sour, and salty foods to help balance their dosha.

On the other hand, someone with a Pitta constitution, associated with heat, intensity, and strong digestion, may benefit from cooling, calming foods like cucumber, coconut water, and mint. They should also avoid spicy or acidic foods and choose naturally sweet, bitter, and astringent foods to balance their dosha.

Therefore, Ayurveda encourages a diet rich in fresh, whole foods appropriate for your constitution and emphasizes the importance of balancing your dosha through food choices to promote overall health and well-being.

Follow a daily routine: Following a daily routine that aligns with your body's natural rhythms can help promote balance and overall well-being. Ayurveda emphasizes the importance of consistency in key areas such as sleep, diet, and relaxation. This may involve waking up and going to bed at the same time every day to help regulate your body's internal clock, eating meals regularly to aid digestion and maintain energy levels, and taking breaks to rest and recharge. Additionally, incorporating meditation or gentle exercise can help reduce stress and promote a sense of calm. Establishing a daily routine for your needs and preferences can help support your physical, mental, and emotional health.

Get enough sleep: Ayurveda emphasizes the importance of adequate sleep for optimal health and well-being. In Ayurveda, sleep is a crucial pillar of health, diet, and exercise.

According to Ayurvedic principles, the body goes through self-repair and rejuvenation during sleep, essential for maintaining physical and mental health. Therefore, getting enough sleep is vital for restoring balance and harmony in the body, promoting a healthy immune system, and reducing the risk of various diseases.

Ayurveda recommends getting 7-8 hours of sleep every night, ideally starting before 10 pm when the body's natural circadian rhythm is in sync with the environment. Going to bed early and waking up early is essential for maintaining overall health and well-being.

In Ayurveda, sleep quality is just as important as quantity. Therefore, Ayurvedic practitioners recommend establishing a relaxing bedtime routine and creating a conducive sleep environment to ensure restful and uninterrupted sleep. Some tips include avoiding stimulating activities before bed, minimizing exposure to electronic devices, and creating a comfortable and peaceful sleep environment.

Practice yoga and meditation: Yoga and meditation are ancient practices used for centuries to promote physical, mental, and spiritual well-being. Yoga involves a series of physical postures and breathing exercises that help increase the body's flexibility, strength, and balance while calming the mind and reducing stress. Meditation, on the other hand, involves focusing the mind on a particular object, thought, or activity to achieve a state of mental clarity and inner peace.

According to Ayurveda, incorporating these practices into your daily routine has numerous health benefits, including reducing stress and anxiety, improving sleep quality, boosting immunity, and promoting overall physical and mental health. Regularly practicing yoga and meditation can increase your body's flexibility, improve your posture, and reduce the risk of developing chronic diseases such as hypertension, diabetes, and heart disease.

In addition to physical health benefits, yoga, and meditation can also help to promote emotional well-being by reducing feelings of depression, anxiety, and stress. These practices can also help to improve cognitive function and enhance mental clarity, making it easier to focus and concentrate on daily tasks.

Use of natural remedies: One of the core principles of Ayurveda is that the body has the ability to heal itself and that natural remedies can be used to support this process.

Ayurvedic remedies often involve herbs, oils, and spices, which are believed to have specific healing properties. For example, ginger tea is a popular Ayurvedic remedy for digestive issues such as nausea, bloating, and indigestion. Ginger contains compounds that can help to stimulate digestion and reduce inflammation in the gut.

Similarly, lavender oil is often used in Ayurvedic aromatherapy to promote relaxation and calm. The scent of lavender has been shown to have a calming effect on the nervous system and can help to reduce feelings of anxiety and stress.

Ayurvedic remedies like turmeric are believed to have anti-inflammatory properties and can treat various conditions, such as joint pain and skin disorders. Holy basil, or tulsi, is another popular Ayurvedic herb believed to have immune-boosting properties and can treat respiratory infections and other illnesses.

Spend time in nature: Ayurveda views humans as integral to the natural world. According to Ayurveda, spending time in nature can help to balance the body, mind, and spirit and promote balance and harmony.

When we spend time in nature, we are exposed to natural elements like fresh air, sunlight, and greenery, which have a therapeutic effect on our bodies and mind. Studies have shown that spending time in nature can reduce stress, lower blood pressure, and improve mood. It can also improve our immunity by exposing us to natural microbes that can help to build our immune system.

Ayurveda recommends various activities to connect with nature, such as walking or hiking, practicing yoga or meditation outdoors, gardening, or simply sitting in a park or by the beach. These activities can help to ground us, promote relaxation, and reduce mental fatigue.

Living in harmony with nature is a fundamental principle in Ayurveda that greatly impacts our overall health and well-being. Adopting lifestyle practices that align with this principle prevents imbalances in our body, mind, and spirit. It's essential to make choices that support our body's natural rhythms and needs to maintain optimal health.

Meditation for emotional stability and self-awareness

Meditation is a practice that has been used for centuries to promote emotional stability and self-awareness. In Ayurveda, an ancient Indian system of medicine, meditation is considered an essential tool for achieving balance and harmony in the mind and body.

Ayurveda teaches that emotions are important to overall health and well-being as they are closely connected to physical and mental health. When our emotions are balanced, we experience a sense of calm, joy, and contentment. However, when our emotions are imbalanced, we may experience stress, anxiety, anger, or other negative emotions. Meditation is considered a powerful way to balance our emotions and prevent these imbalances.

Meditation is a powerful tool for balancing emotions and promoting emotional stability. It is a mental practice that involves training the mind to focus and be present in the current moment without judgment, which helps to reduce stress and anxiety. Regular meditation practice can help us develop greater self-awareness and a deeper understanding of our emotions and how they affect us. This, in turn, can lead to greater emotional stability and a more balanced state of mind.

When we observe moments without reacting or judging them, we learn to regulate our emotional responses and become less reactive to challenging situations. As a result, we become more aware of our thoughts and emotions, allowing us to identify patterns and triggers that may be causing us to experience negative emotions. This self-awareness can also help us develop greater empathy for others and improve our relationships with them.

Ayurveda recommends various meditation techniques to balance the Mahagunas, including mindfulness, mantra, and pranayama (breathing exercises). The specific technique chosen will depend on the individual's constitution and needs. If you have a Vata dosha, meditation techniques that focus on grounding and stability will be beneficial for you. On the other hand, if you have a Pitta dosha, cooling and calming techniques will be more helpful. To determine the best meditation practice for your needs, it is recommended to consult an Ayurvedic practitioner.

Mantra meditation involves repeating a specific sound or word. "OM" is the sacred sound or chant used in the Hindu tradition while focusing the mind on the sound and the vibrations it creates in the body. The mantra's delicate repetition allows the mind to experience increasingly subtler levels of the thought process until thought and emotion are transcended. Another very powerful mantra is Alaha, a sacred Aramaic name of the Divine Creator used to open and vibrate the heart and unfold the wisdom of Ayurveda within you. The frequent use of sacred sounds applied after daily prayer or meditation practice is believed to help balance the doshas and promote emotional stability. The mantra's objective is to provide a vehicle for the mind to transcend and opens a door to witness the state of the heart.

Another popular meditation practice in Ayurveda is mindfulness meditation. This involves focusing the mind on the present moment and observing thoughts and emotions without judgment. By practicing mindfulness regularly, we can develop greater self-awareness and learn to respond to emotions more balanced and mindfully.

In addition to promoting emotional balance, meditation is also believed to have a range of other health benefits, according to Ayurveda, including improved concentration, better sleep, and reduced stress.

Sufi chants or sound healing are power mantra for meditation and sound healing. They vibrate the heart to release negative emotions, pain, and veils, and they promote calmness and deep relaxation of the heart, mind, and body.

Ayurveda emphasizes the importance of developing a regular meditation practice to experience these benefits. Even a few minutes of meditation each day can help calm the mind and promote emotional stability, making it an accessible and effective tool for anyone looking to improve their health and well-being. Meditation is the most effective method for achieving internal change. Through regular meditation, we secure the systematic practice of self-referral and link our awareness with the intellect that sustains and regulates the universe. Meditation is an energy agent that assists us in maintaining emotional stability and self-awareness.

Here are some steps to help you get started:

- Find a quiet place where you won't be disturbed. Sit comfortably with your back straight and your hands resting on your lap.
- Focus on your breath. Close your eyes and take a few deep breaths. Then, breathe naturally and focus on the sensation of the breath moving in and out of your body.

- Notice when your mind wanders. As you focus on your breath, you may notice that your mind starts to wander; this is normal. When you notice your mind is wandering, gently bring your awareness back to your breath, bow your head to your heart, feel your chest expanding and vibrating as you chant a mantra.
- Practice self-compassion. Meditation can be challenging, especially when you're first starting. Be patient, and don't judge yourself harshly if you find it difficult to focus.
- Set a timer. Start with a short meditation, such as five or ten minutes, and gradually increase the length of your meditation sessions over time.

- Consider guided meditation. If you find it difficult to meditate on your own, try using a guided meditation app or video. These resources can help you stay focused and guide you in meditating effectively.

- Be consistent. The more you practice meditation, the easier it will become. Aim to meditate for a few minutes every day, even if it's just for a few minutes. Consistency is key to developing emotional stability and self-awareness through meditation.

Remember that meditation is a skill that takes time to develop. With regular practice, you can develop greater emotional stability and self-awareness, which can help you navigate life's challenges more easily and clearly.

Dinacharya (daily regimen)

Dinacharya, which translates to daily routine in Sanskrit, is a powerful tool for achieving balance and promoting overall health. Our daily habits significantly impact our well-being, and a consistent routine is more effective than occasional remedies in maintaining health. By aligning our daily activities with the natural cycles of the day, Dinacharya establishes healthy patterns and supports the body's natural healing potential.

The three doshas - Vata, Pitta, and Kapha - have distinct periods of dominance within a twenty-four-hour cycle. Establishing a daily routine that aligns with these natural cycles promotes balance and harmony within the body and mind. This may involve waking up and going to bed consistently, eating meals at regular intervals, and engaging in appropriate activities for each time of day. Regular practice of Dinacharya supports our body's natural healing potential and cultivates a deeper sense of well-being.

Dinacharya Cycles

According to Ayurveda, the ancient Indian system of medicine, our daily routine should be aligned with the natural cycles of the sun and the moon, which are believed to influence our bodily functions and energy levels. Ayurveda divides the day into two cycles: the solar cycle, which begins at sunrise and ends at sunset, and the lunar cycle, which begins at sunset and ends at sunrise.

Within each cycle, four-hour periods are dominated by different doshas, or energies, known as Vata, Pitta, and Kapha. These doshas are present in everyone's body, but their proportions vary from person to person, determining their Ayurvedic body type.

These cycles are as follows:

Vata Time (2 am - 6 am): This time is dominated by the Vata dosha, which is associated with movement and activity. During this time, the body is naturally waking up, and it is recommended to wake up early in the morning, around 4-5 am to take advantage of the Vata time. During this time, one should perform self-care practices or Dinacharya practices, meditation, or prayer.

Kapha Time (6 am - 10 am): This time is dominated by the Kapha dosha, which is associated with stability and nourishment. During this time, the digestive system is at its peak, and it is recommended to eat a healthy breakfast to nourish the body. This is also a good time for exercise, as the Kapha dosha provides strength and stability.

Pitta Time (10 am - 2 pm): This time is dominated by the pitta dosha, which is associated with metabolism and transformation. During this time, the digestive system is still active, and it is recommended to have a heavy lunch. This is also a good time for mental work and creative activities.

Vata Time (2 pm - 6 pm): This time is dominated by the Vata dosha again, and it is a good time for socializing, creative activities, and exercise. One should avoid heavy meals during this time, as the digestive system is less active.

Kapha Time (6 pm - 10 pm): This time is dominated by the Kapha dosha again, and it is recommended to have a light dinner during this time. One should avoid mental stimulation and instead relax and unwind.

Pitta Time (10 pm - 2 am): This time is dominated by the Pitta dosha again, and it is recommended to go to bed early, around

10 pm. The body is naturally winding down, and it is important to get enough rest during this time.

Dinacharya Ayurveda Practices

Dinacharya involves a set of practices that should be performed daily to maintain good health. These practices are as follows:

Waking: Waking up early is an essential Dinacharya practice and can help us cultivate a sense of purpose and fulfillment. It helps align our body with the natural circadian rhythm and promotes good health. If there are time constraints, taking a few deep breaths and adopting an attitude of gratitude for waking up to a new day can help set a positive tone for the day ahead. Additionally, waking up early allows us to establish a routine and create the positive qualities of alertness, vibrancy, enthusiasm, energy, clarity, strengthened intuition, and motivation, which can promote balance and harmony in the body and mind.

Elimination: Regular elimination is crucial for maintaining good health in Ayurveda. It includes practices like bowel movements and urination. You should try to have a bowel movement simultaneously every day and avoid holding it in. Drinking warm water and herbal teas and incorporating fibrous foods in your diet can help regulate bowel movements. Similarly, urination should be regular, and you should avoid holding it in for long periods. This simple practice also enkindles agni, the digestive fire essential for proper digestion and assimilation of nutrients. Proper elimination is crucial for maintaining optimal health and preventing many imbalances in the body. Therefore, it is essential to establish a routine of eliminating waste products from the body, which helps to keep the digestive system healthy and promotes overall well-being. Drinking warm water with lemon in the morning is an effective way to kickstart this process and support a healthy digestive system.

Cleansing the senses: Purifying the senses is essential to prepare the mind and body for a new day filled with rich experiences. Purifying the senses involves refreshing and energizing the mind by performing a series of simple yet effective rituals. This includes practices like oil pulling, neti pot, and eye cleansing. Oil pulling involves swishing warm sesame oil in your mouth for a few minutes to remove toxins and promote oral health. Neti pot uses a saline solution to cleanse the nasal passages, while eye cleansing involves using rosewater or Triphala to rinse the eyes.

Abhyanga: Abhyanga involves massaging warm oil onto the body, which nourishes and strengthens the body, calms the mind, and encourages regular sleep patterns. It also stimulates the internal organs, enhances blood circulation, and can significantly reduce Vata dosha, which is responsible for many imbalances in the body. The practice of Abhyanga should be done daily to experience its full benefits. It is recommended to use warm, herbal oils specific to your dosha for maximum effectiveness. The massage should be gentle yet firm, starting from the extremities and moving toward the heart. Sesame oil is commonly used for Abhyanga, but coconut or almond oil can also be used. Regular Abhyanga can help promote balance and harmony in the body and mind, leading to overall well-being.

Clothing: Dinacharya emphasizes the importance of wearing clean clothing from natural fibers like cotton, wool, linen, or silk. It is believed that these fabrics help maintain the body's energy balance and provide comfort. However, wearing used clothing, especially other people's shoes, is discouraged in Ayurveda because they can carry negative subtle energies that can disrupt the body's natural energy flow.

Therefore, choosing new and fresh clothing and avoiding sharing personal items like footwear is recommended to maintain a positive and healthy energy balance in the body. Additionally, regularly washing and airing out clothes is essential for keeping them clean and fresh, promoting good hygiene and overall well-being.

Take your herbs: In the ancient Ayurvedic practice of Dinacharya, taking herbs is an important aspect of daily self-care. To enhance herbs' medicinal effect, taking them simultaneously each day is recommended, ideally during your morning routine. This consistent timing allows the body to develop a natural rhythm and better absorb the herbs over time.

When it comes to taking herbs, it's important to consider the timing of meals. Herbs taken on an empty stomach are the most potent action in the body because the digestive system is not preoccupied with food processing. This allows the herbs to be quickly absorbed and distributed throughout the body, promoting their medicinal effects.

However, it's important to exercise caution when taking certain herbs on an empty stomach, as they may cause stomach irritation or discomfort. In these cases, taking the herbs with a small meal or snack may be best.

Meditation: In today's fast-paced world, taking care of our mental well-being is essential, just like we take care of our physical health. Practicing meditation is one of the most effective ways to achieve this. Meditation lets us cleanse our minds of negative thoughts and emotions hindering our growth and progress. Staying still and directing our attention inward helps us better understand ourselves and our surroundings. Focusing on our breath and practicing pranayama can enable us to control our thoughts and emotions, leading to a more peaceful and relaxed mind. Even with limited time, setting aside just twenty minutes for meditation or inviting calm and relaxation into the body can benefit significantly. Meditation can provide a protective shield against the destabilizing effects of the external environment, allowing us to remain grounded and centered when facing challenges. Regular meditation can help us develop inner strength and resilience, ultimately leading to a more satisfying and meaningful life.

Aerobic exercise: According to Ayurveda, engaging in regular aerobic exercise is beneficial for improving cardiovascular health and stamina. Ayurvedic principles suggest that the period between dawn and 10 am is dominated by the Kapha dosha, characterized by heaviness, slowness, and stability. The longer one stays in bed after sunrise, the more Kapha qualities will be in their physiology throughout the day. Therefore, this period is ideal for engaging in more physical activities like jogging, swimming, or cycling that help to counterbalance the Kapha qualities. Specifically, between 7 am to 10 am is considered the most optimal time for aerobic exercise as it helps to stimulate the metabolism, boost energy levels, and invigorate the body and mind for the day ahead. Engaging in these activities during this period can also help to improve overall physical fitness, mental clarity, and emotional well-being.

Work and lunch: Ayurveda recommends that the most productive time for work is from 10 am to 2 pm when the sun is at its peak and the digestive fire is strong. Eating the largest meal of the day during this time is ideal to ensure efficient digestion, assimilation, and metabolism of nutrients. This increases energy, strength, and alertness and reduces the desire for snacking and overeating. Taking a short stroll after lunch can aid digestion.

Creative work: Engaging in creative work like painting, writing, or music can help stimulate the mind and reduce stress. Vata is an excellent time to engage in creative work. At this time, Vata types may experience a drop in energy and would benefit from a modest snack.

Evening meal: Ayurveda recommends having a light, early dinner that is easy to digest. Evening meals should contain light foods like toast, rice, milk beverages, noodles, and soup. You must wait at least 4 hours after your previous meal to ensure proper digestion. Ideally, the evening meal should be eaten before sunset and at least three hours before bedtime. Avoiding heavy, greasy, or spicy foods can help promote good digestion and a night of restful sleep.

Relaxation: Taking time to relax and unwind is essential in Ayurveda. You can practice relaxation techniques like deep breathing, meditation, or gentle yoga. Before bedtime, it is recommended to unwind and relax during the Kapha period in the evening. For restful sleep, it is essential to be in bed before this dosha reaches its maximum. To relax, enjoy activities such as reading or listening to soothing music. Taking triphala tea a half-hour before bedtime can help to restore the digestive system.

Bathing: In Ayurveda, bathing is considered a therapeutic part of personal hygiene that helps to relax muscles and remove dirt, sweat, and other impurities from the body, which can lead to the accumulation of toxins. Ayurveda recommends bathing in the morning, as it can help to refresh and energize the body for the day ahead. It is also important to use lukewarm water to avoid overstimulating the skin and aggravating Vata dosha.

Additionally, Ayurveda recommends incorporating certain herbs or oils into the bathing routine to enhance its therapeutic benefits. For example, using neem leaves in the water can help to purify the skin, while adding a few drops of lavender oil can have a calming effect on the mind.

Sleep: Getting an adequate and restful night's sleep is crucial for our health, and it's important to be aware of the body's natural cycles. Ayurveda recommends going to bed early and waking up early, as this is considered the most conducive time for restful sleep. The Pitta period, from 10 pm to 2 am, is when the body needs rest to eliminate toxins and impurities. Going to bed by 10 pm will ensure 6-7 hours of refreshing sleep.

In addition to the duration of sleep, Ayurveda also emphasizes the quality of sleep. This includes creating a peaceful sleeping environment, such as keeping the bedroom dark, quiet, and comfortable. Avoiding stimulating activities like using electronic devices, watching TV, or working before bed is also important.

To ensure a good night's sleep, it may be helpful to apply oil to your scalp and feet before going to bed. While you sleep, your body processes the food you ate during the day, but it may struggle with larger or heavier meals. For this reason, it is suggested to choose lighter, easy-to-digest meals for the evening.

Benefits of Dinacharya (daily regimen)

The benefits of Dinacharya are numerous and can positively impact every aspect of one's life. Here are some of the benefits of following a daily regimen:

Boosts immunity: Dinacharya helps to strengthen the immune system and protect the body against diseases and infections.

Improves digestion: Following a daily regimen can improve digestion, help in better absorption of nutrients, and prevent digestive disorders like constipation and indigestion.

Enhances sleep quality: A consistent daily routine can help regulate the body's circadian rhythm, leading to better quality sleep and improved overall health.

Reduces stress: A daily regimen can help reduce stress and anxiety, improving mental health and overall well-being.

Promotes self-discipline: Dinacharya promotes self-discipline and helps to establish healthy habits, which can be beneficial in achieving personal and professional goals.

Enhances productivity: Establishing a routine can increase productivity and efficiency, leading to better performance in all areas of life.

Improves skin and hair health: Dinacharya includes practices like oil massage, which can improve skin and hair health, making them appear more vibrant and youthful.

Ritucharya (seasonal regimen)

Ritucharya is a concept in Ayurveda that refers to the seasonal regimen or lifestyle practices followed to maintain optimal health and wellness throughout the year. Ayurveda recognizes that each season has a unique effect on the body and mind; therefore, specific practices are recommended to balance the effects of each season.

The year is divided into six seasons in Ayurveda - Vasanta (spring), Greeshma (summer), Varsha (monsoon), Sharada (autumn), Hemanta (winter), and Shishira (late winter). Here are some general guidelines for each season:

Vasanta (Spring): Spring is characterized by the Kapha dosha (one of the three doshas in Ayurveda) and is a time of renewal and rejuvenation. Ayurveda recommends consuming light, warm, and dry foods and engaging in activities that promote movement and physical exercise. A dry massage with herbal powders or oils is also recommended.

Greeshma (Summer): Summer is characterized by the Pitta dosha when the digestive fire is strong. Ayurveda recommends consuming cooling, hydrating foods and beverages like fruits, salads, and coconut water. It is also important to protect oneself from the sun and to avoid excessive physical activity during the hottest parts of the day.

Varsha (Monsoon): Monsoon is characterized by the Vata dosha, a time when the body's digestive fire is weakened. Ayurveda recommends consuming light, easily digestible foods and avoiding heavy, oily, or fried foods. It is also important to keep oneself warm and dry and to avoid getting wet in the rain.

Sharada (Autumn): Autumn is characterized by the Vata dosha and is a time of change and transition. Ayurveda recommends consuming warm, nourishing foods and engaging in activities that promote relaxation, such as yoga and meditation. It is also important to protect oneself from the cold and wind.

Hemanta (Winter): Winter is characterized by the Vata dosha when the body's digestive fire is strong. Ayurveda recommends consuming warm, nourishing foods and engaging in activities that promote physical exercise and movement. Dry massage with herbal oils is also recommended.

Shishira (Late Winter): Late winter is characterized by the Kapha dosha and is a time of congestion and stagnation. Ayurveda recommends consuming light, warm, and dry foods and engaging in activities that promote movement and physical exercise. A dry massage with herbal powders or oils is also recommended.

In addition to these general guidelines, Ayurveda also recommends specific practices and treatments for each individual, depending on their unique constitution and current state of health. It is important to consult with an Ayurvedic practitioner to determine the most appropriate Ritucharya regimen for you.

Balancing doshas with the help of opposites

Ayurvedic texts emphasize the importance of balance in achieving optimal health and well-being. According to this ancient system of medicine, each person has a unique constitution of varying proportions of the three doshas - Vata, Pitta, and Kapha. When these doshas are balanced, a person experiences good health, vitality, and emotional balance. However, there is a correlation between physical and mental health imbalances and various health issues that can arise.

To maintain balance, Ayurveda teaches that it is necessary to be aware of the 20 common qualities or attributes experienced throughout nature. These qualities are known as "guna" in Sanskrit and are categorized into ten pairs of opposites. The ten pairs of opposites are:

1. Heavy (Guru) / Light (Laghu)
2. Oily (Snigdha) / Dry (Ruksha)
3. Cold (Shita) / Hot (Ushna)
4. Dull (Manda) / Sharp (Tikshna)
5. Soft (Mrudu) / Hard (Kathina)
6. Slow (Manda) / Fast (Tivra)
7. Stable (Sthira) / Mobile (Chala)
8. Gross (Sthula) / Subtle (Sukshma)
9. Smooth (Sara) / Rough (Khara)
10. Dense (Sandra) / Liquid (Drava)

Ayurveda teaches that too much or too little of any one quality can disrupt the balance of the doshas and cause health issues. Therefore, when an individual is experiencing an imbalance in their doshas, they are advised to seek the opposite quality for healing. For example, suppose a person is experiencing excess heat in their body due to an imbalance in the Pitta dosha. In that case, they should seek cooling and calming foods and activities to balance the excess heat.

Understanding the qualities or attributes of nature and using their opposites to balance the doshas is a cornerstone of Ayurvedic medicine. Practicing this principle can help individuals achieve greater physical and emotional balance, leading to a healthier and happier life.

Here are some examples of how the 20 qualities can be used based on the 3 doshas:

Vata Dosha: Vata is characterized by dryness, coldness, lightness, and mobility. To balance Vata, you should consume foods and engage in activities that are opposite in nature, such as:

- Consuming warm, moist, and nourishing foods
- Drinking warm fluids
- Engaging in regular physical exercise but avoiding excessive activity
- Getting enough rest and sleep
- Practicing grounding and calming activities like yoga, meditation, and deep breathing exercises

Pitta Dosha: Pitta is characterized by heat, intensity, and sharpness. To balance Pitta, you should consume foods and engage in activities that are opposite in nature, such as:

- Consuming cool, refreshing, and hydrating foods
- Drinking plenty of water and herbal teas
- Engaging in moderate physical exercise but avoiding excessive heat or intensity
- Getting enough rest and avoiding overworking
- Practicing relaxation and cooling activities like swimming, walking in nature, and massage therapy

Kapha Dosha: Kapha is characterized by heaviness, coldness, and stability. To balance Kapha, you should consume foods and engage in activities that are opposite in nature, such as:

- Consuming warm, light, and spicy foods
- Drinking warm fluids, avoiding cold drinks

- Engaging in regular physical exercise, with emphasis on cardio and strength training
- Getting enough stimulation and avoiding stagnation
- Practicing invigorating and energizing activities like dancing, hiking, and cardio exercises.

Please note that keeping your doshas in balance is an ongoing process that requires constant attention and commitment. We suggest seeking guidance from an Ayurvedic practitioner to discover your specific dosha constitution and receive personalized recommendations for lifestyle practices and remedies that will help you maintain balance.

Listening to your inner wisdom (concept of Prajnaparadha—one of the three fundamental causes of disease)

Ayurveda, the ancient Indian system of medicine, has long recognized the interconnectedness of physical, mental, and spiritual well-being. It emphasizes that good health is not merely the absence of disease but a complete physical, mental, and spiritual balance. To achieve this state, Ayurveda emphasizes the importance of balancing the three doshas, maintaining a healthy digestive system, and living in harmony with nature. However, one of the fundamental causes of disease that is often overlooked is Prajnaparadha, or the "crime against wisdom."

Prajnaparadha is the act of ignoring or suppressing our inner wisdom or intuition. According to Ayurvedic philosophy, every individual has an innate wisdom or intelligence that guides them toward optimal health and well-being. This wisdom is connected to the universe's larger intelligence and is accessed through intuition, inner knowing, and gut feelings.

In today's fast-paced and stressful world, it is easy to become disconnected from our inner wisdom and rely solely on external sources of information and guidance. We often make choices that do not align with our true nature, resulting in toxins and imbalances in the body, mind, and spirit. Over time, this can lead to the manifestation of diseases and other health issues.

To avoid Prajnaparadha and promote optimal health, Ayurveda recommends cultivating awareness and mindfulness of our thoughts, emotions, and actions. It involves tuning into our inner voice and trusting our intuition. Practicing meditation, yoga, and other mindfulness practices can help us connect with our inner wisdom and intuition. These practices can help us learn to listen to our bodies, observe our thoughts and feelings, and make choices that align with our true nature.

In addition to physical health, Prajnaparadha can also affect our mental and emotional health. Ignoring our inner wisdom and intuition can lead to feelings of dissatisfaction, anxiety, and depression and can impact our relationships and overall quality of life.

Ayurveda teaches us that our inner wisdom is a valuable tool for promoting optimal health and well-being. By learning to listen to our intuition and making choices that align with our true nature, we can prevent the accumulation of toxins and imbalances and support our overall health and well-being. In addition, we can improve our mental and emotional health and experience a greater sense of peace, joy, and fulfillment in our lives.

Enjoying optimal health and vitality by maximizing the finest essences of doshas: Ojas, Tejas, Prana (definition, how they influence you, how to increase them)

Ayurveda recognizes that maintaining optimal health and vitality is not just about balancing the three doshas - Vata, Pitta, and Kapha. Three subtle essences of these doshas are crucial in promoting overall well-being - Ojas, Tejas, and Prana.

Ojas and how it influences you

Ojas is a subtle essence of Kapha dosha and is considered one of the finest essences of doshas in Ayurveda. It is the ultimate product of healthy digestion and represents the essence of all body tissues, including the immune system. Ojas is responsible for maintaining immunity and vitality in the body and plays a crucial role in maintaining overall health and well-being. Below are ways in which Ojas can influence you:

Boosts Immunity: Ojas maintains the immune system, which is essential for fighting infections and diseases. When Ojas is abundant, an individual possesses radiant health and a strong immune system. On the other hand, when Ojas is depleted, an individual may experience fatigue, weakness, and susceptibility to disease.

Promotes Radiant Skin: Ojas contributes to healthy and glowing skin. A sufficient amount of Ojas gives the skin a radiant appearance and the individual a healthy and vibrant look. On the other hand, if Ojas is lacking, the skin may appear dull, dry, and lifeless.

Enhances Energy Levels: Ojas is responsible for providing energy to the body. When Ojas is abundant, an individual feels energetic and lively. On the other hand, when Ojas is depleted, an individual may experience fatigue, lethargy, and a lack of energy.

Increases Mental Clarity: Ojas also enhances mental clarity and cognitive function. When Ojas is abundant, an individual has a clear, focused mind and can think and concentrate better. When the Ojas of a person is low, they may encounter difficulties in focusing, experiencing mental fogginess, and confusion.

Promotes Emotional Well-being: Ojas is also responsible for promoting emotional well-being. When Ojas is abundant, an individual feels happy, content, and emotionally stable. In contrast, when Ojas is minimal, an individual may experience mood swings, anxiety, and depression.

Enhances Reproductive Health: Ojas is responsible for maintaining reproductive health in both men and women. When Ojas is abundant, it enhances fertility, improves sexual function, and increase libido. In contrast, when Ojas is depleted, it can lead to infertility, impotence, and decreased libido.

Supports Longevity: Ojas has benefits for longevity and overall lifespan. Having an abundance of Ojas can protect the body from aging, resulting in a longer and healthier life. On the other hand, if Ojas is low, it can lead to premature aging and a shorter life.

How to increase Ojas

Here are some ways to increase Ojas:

Eat nutrient-dense foods: Ayurveda recommends consuming foods rich in vitamins, minerals, and antioxidants to nourish the body and increase Ojas. Fresh fruits and vegetables, whole grains, nuts, seeds, and healthy fats like ghee and coconut oil are all excellent choices.

Practice mindfulness and self-care: Stress and negative emotions can deplete Ojas. Therefore, engaging in self-care practices that promote relaxation and reduce stress is essential. This may include meditation, yoga, massage, and aromatherapy.

Get adequate rest: Quality sleep is vital for the body to restore and rejuvenate itself. Ayurveda recommends getting at least 7-8 hours of sleep each night to support the production of Ojas.

Engage in activities that promote happiness and joy: Doing things that make you happy and bring you joy can help to increase Ojas. This may include spending time with loved ones, engaging in creative activities, or pursuing hobbies that bring you fulfillment.

Practice pranayama: Pranayama, or breathing exercises, can help increase Ojas by improving oxygenation and promoting relaxation. Slow, deep breathing exercises such as Nadi Shodhana (alternate nostril breathing) and Ujjayi breathing are especially effective.

Avoid excessive physical and mental exertion: Over-exertion can deplete Ojas, so balancing physical activity with relaxation is important. Over-stimulating the mind with excessive mental activity or exposure to technology can also deplete Ojas. Taking breaks from screens and engaging in activities that promote mental relaxation can help to prevent this.

Tejas and how it influences you

Tejas is one of the three Doshas or essential life energies in our body according to Ayurveda, the ancient Indian system of medicine. It is characterized as the force of transformation and is responsible for digestion, metabolism, and the body's ability to transform food into energy. Tejas is also considered the source of mental and physical prowess and is responsible for maintaining our inner strength, radiance, and vitality. When Tejas is balanced, an individual possesses a sharp mind, strong willpower, and the ability to make sound decisions. However, when Tejas is imbalanced, an individual may experience mental fog, confusion, and lack of motivation.

Here are some ways that Tejas can influence you:

Digestion and metabolism: Tejas is responsible for the digestive fire or **agni,** which is essential for the digestion and metabolism of food. A healthy balance of Tejas helps to ensure that our food is properly digested and assimilated, while an imbalance can lead to digestive problems like acid reflux, bloating, and constipation.

Skin health: Tejas is responsible for the luster and glow of the skin. A healthy Tejas balance helps keep the skin soft, smooth, and radiant, while an imbalance can lead to skin problems like acne, rashes, and dryness.

Vision and eye health: Tejas is located primarily in the eyes and is responsible for the sharpness of vision. A healthy balance of Tejas helps keep the eyes healthy and clear, while an imbalance can lead to problems like dry eyes, eye strain, and poor vision.

Mental clarity and focus: Tejas is closely related to intelligence and mental clarity. A healthy balance of Tejas helps to keep the mind sharp and focused, while an imbalance can lead to mental fog, confusion, and forgetfulness.

Courage and ambition: Tejas is associated with courage, willpower, and ambition. A healthy balance of Tejas helps to promote these qualities, while an imbalance can lead to a lack of motivation, procrastination, and fearfulness.

Emotional balance: Tejas is also responsible for emotional balance and stability. It helps to regulate emotions and prevents excessive mood swings.

How to increase Tejas

If you have a low Tejas level, there are several things you can do to increase it. Here are some tips for increasing Tejas:

Eat a balanced and healthy diet: A balanced diet that includes fresh fruits and vegetables, whole grains, lean proteins, and healthy fats is important for increasing Tejas. Foods that are rich in antioxidants and nutrients like vitamins A, C, and E can help to promote healthy skin and vision. Avoid processed foods, sugary drinks, excessive amounts of caffeine, alcohol, and spicy or fried foods.

Practice yoga and pranayama: Yoga and pranayama are ancient practices that can help to increase Tejas. Yoga postures that focus on the solar plexus, such as boat pose (Navasana), and pranayama techniques like Kapalabhati and Bhastrika can help to stimulate the digestive fire and promote mental clarity.

Get regular exercise: Exercise is important for promoting digestion, circulation, and mental clarity, all associated with Tejas. Try incorporating regular exercise into your routine, such as brisk walking, jogging, or cycling. You can also try more energetic exercises like dancing, martial arts, or team sports.

Practice meditation: Meditation is a powerful tool for increasing Tejas. Regular meditation can help promote mental clarity, reduce stress, and enhance focus and purpose. There are many different types of meditation, including mindfulness, vipassana, and guided imagery.

Spend time in nature: Spending time in nature is beneficial for increasing Tejas. It can reduce stress, promote relaxation, and improve your overall well-being. Make it a point to spend time outdoors daily, such as walking in the park, hiking in the mountains, or swimming in a natural body of water.

Practice self-care: Self-care is an important part of increasing Tejas. Take time each day to do things that nourish your body and mind, such as taking a warm bath, getting a massage, or reading a good book. Avoid overworking and overextending yourself and make time for relaxation and leisure activities.

Use aromatherapy: Essential oils like sandalwood, rose, and frankincense can help to increase Tejas. You can use these oils in a diffuser or add a few drops to a warm bath or massage oil. These oils can help promote mental clarity, reduce stress, and enhance well-being.

Prana and how it influences you

The term "Prana" comes from Sanskrit and means "life force" or "vital energy." It is a subtle essence present in all living beings and is responsible for sustaining life through breath. Prana is considered one of the finest essences of the doshas, and it plays a vital role in maintaining health and well-being. It is responsible for the proper functioning of the respiratory system, the circulation of blood, and the elimination of waste from the body. Prana also influences the mind, emotions, and consciousness. When Prana is abundant, an individual is said to possess high levels of energy and creativity and a deep connection to their inner self. However, when Prana is imbalanced, an individual may experience fatigue, apathy, and a lack of inspiration.

Here are some ways in which Prana influences you:

Respiration: Prana is responsible for the proper functioning of the respiratory system. It governs the intake of oxygen and the elimination of carbon dioxide from the body. When Prana is balanced, breathing is smooth and effortless, and the body can take in the required amount of oxygen.

Circulation: The circulation of blood in our body is controlled by Prana. This regulates the transportation of oxygen and nutrients to the cells and tissues and helps eliminate waste products. When Prana is balanced, our body can maintain optimal health, and blood circulation remains smooth.

Digestion: Prana also influences the digestive system. It governs the secretion of digestive juices and enzymes and food movement through the digestive tract. When the balance of

Prana is maintained, the body's digestion becomes efficient, and it can properly absorb nutrients.

Emotional and mental state: Prana also influences the mind and emotions. It governs the body's energy flow and the nervous system's balance. When Prana is balanced, the mind and emotions are clear.

Consciousness: Prana is also responsible for consciousness. It governs the state of awareness and the ability to perceive and respond to the environment. When Prana is balanced, consciousness is clear, and the individual can experience the world fully.

How to increase Prana

There are several ways to increase Prana in the body. Some of these ways include:

Pranayama: Pranayama is a yogic practice that involves breathing exercises to increase Prana in the body. These exercises include Nadi Shodhana, Kapalabhati, and Bhramari Pranayama.

Yoga: Yoga is another practice that can increase Prana in the body. Different yoga poses and asanas help balance and regulate Prana's flow throughout the body.

Meditation: Meditation is a practice that can increase Prana by calming the mind and reducing stress. When the mind is calm, the Prana can flow more freely through the body.

Diet: Eating a healthy, balanced diet can also increase Prana in the body. Fresh fruits and vegetables, whole grains, and lean proteins can give the body the essential nutrients needed to maintain optimal health and well-being.

Sunlight: Spending time in the sunlight can also increase Prana in the body. Sunlight provides the body with vitamin D, essential for maintaining a healthy immune system and balancing the flow of Prana.

Nature walks: Walking in nature can also increase Prana in the body. The fresh air, greenery, and natural environment can help to reduce stress and balance the flow of Prana throughout the body.

Massage: Massaging the body can also increase Prana by promoting relaxation and reducing muscle tension. This can help to improve the flow of Prana throughout the body.

Sound therapy: Listening to calming music or chanting can increase Prana in the body through sound therapy. The vibrations and sounds produced can balance and regulate the flow of Prana throughout the body.

Positive thinking: Positive thinking and affirmations can also increase Prana by promoting a positive mindset and reducing stress and negative emotions.

In conclusion, Ayurveda emphasizes maximizing the subtle essences of doshas - Ojas, Tejas, and Prana - to achieve optimal health and vitality. By increasing these subtle essences, individuals can promote overall well-being, enhance immunity, improve mental clarity, and achieve a deeper connection with their inner self. Ayurvedic principles can help individuals cultivate a balanced and harmonious relationship with their body, mind, and spirit, leading to a healthier and more fulfilling life.

Reducing ama buildup

In Ayurveda, "ama" refers to toxic substances that build up in the body due to poor digestion, metabolism, and elimination. This buildup can cause various health problems, including fatigue, joint pain, inflammation, depression, frequent illness, indecisiveness, and digestive issues. It's essential to reduce ama buildup to maintain optimal health and well-being.

Here are some ways to reduce ama buildup in the body:

Follow a healthy diet: Eating a healthy diet reduces ama buildup. Avoid processed foods, fried foods, and heavy meats, and instead focus on fresh fruits and vegetables, whole grains, and lean proteins.

Drink plenty of water: Drinking plenty of water can help flush toxins out of the body and reduce ama buildup. Aim for at least eight glasses of water a day.

Practice mindful eating: Mindful eating involves paying attention to your food and eating slowly and consciously. This can help improve digestion and reduce ama buildup.

Exercise regularly: Regular exercise can help improve digestion, metabolism, and elimination, which can help reduce ama buildup in the body.

Practice daily detoxification: Practicing daily detoxification practices such as oil pulling, tongue scraping, and dry brushing can help reduce ama buildup in the body.

Get enough sleep: Getting enough sleep is crucial for proper digestion and elimination, which can help reduce ama buildup in the body. Aim for seven to eight hours of sleep each night.

Manage stress: Stress can disrupt digestion and metabolism, leading to ama buildup. Practicing stress-reducing techniques such as yoga, meditation, or deep breathing can help reduce ama buildup in the body.

Take Ayurvedic herbs: Ayurvedic herbs such as triphala, ginger, and turmeric can help improve digestion and reduce ama buildup in the body. Consult an Ayurvedic practitioner to determine which herbs are best for your needs.

In conclusion, reducing ama buildup in the body is crucial for maintaining optimal health and well-being. By following a healthy diet, drinking plenty of water, practicing mindful eating, exercising regularly, practicing daily detoxification, getting enough sleep, managing stress, and taking Ayurvedic herbs, you can reduce ama buildup in the body and promote overall health and wellness.

Panchakarma and Rasayana

Ayurveda encompasses two significant branches, namely Panchakarma and Rasayana. Panchakarma, which translates to "five actions," is a detoxification therapy that aims to remove toxins and impurities from the body through specific techniques. On the other hand, Rasayana, which means "rejuvenation," focuses on promoting longevity and vitality by restoring the balance of the body and mind. These therapies have been practiced for thousands of years and are widely used today to improve overall health and well-being. When combined, Panchakarma and Rasayana offer a powerful tool for individuals to achieve a healthier and more balanced physical and mental state.

Panchakarma as a detoxification therapy

Panchakarma is a unique branch of Ayurveda that has been practiced for thousands of years and used to cleanse the body of toxins and restore its natural balance. It is not only used for enhancing health and well-being but also for rectifying long-standing chronic diseases. The word 'Panchakarma' means 'five actions' in Sanskrit, referring to five different treatments that work together to purify the body and restore its natural balance. The treatment aims to rejuvenate and revitalize the mind and body by systematically strengthening and balancing all the major tissues and organs using a wide range of therapeutic measures.

In the modern era, many people are turning to herbal concoctions, coffee enemas, and colonic irrigation to detoxify their bodies. However, these methods are often only partially successful as they only target limited body organs and fail to treat the body in an integrated way. They tend to help eliminate water-based toxins only, leaving the more resistant and potentially disease-causing oil-based toxins behind.

Panchakarma treatment is unique in its ability to eliminate water effectively- and oil-based toxins from the body, thus helping to rejuvenate and revitalize the whole body. Through therapeutic procedures tailored to the client's constitution or imbalance (prakriti), Panchakarma systematically helps to release, melt, loosen, mobilize, and eliminate toxins and impurities from all the bodily tissues.

The treatment begins with a consultation to determine the client's constitution and any imbalances in their body. Based on this information, a customized treatment plan is created that includes a combination of therapeutic measures, such as massage, herbal steam therapy, enemas, and other techniques, to help eliminate toxins from the body.

The Panchakarma treatment process includes three stages: Purva Karma (preparatory procedures), Pradhana Karma (main procedures), and Paschat Karma (post-procedure care). During the Purva Karma stage, the client undergoes preparatory procedures to help loosen and mobilize toxins in the body. In the Pradhana Karma stage, the main Panchakarma procedures are performed to eliminate toxins from the body. Finally, post-procedure care is given in the Paschat Karma stage to help the client's body and mind rejuvenate.

After cleansing the tissues and strengthening the digestive fire, our bodies can effectively metabolize the food and herbs we consume. This leads to improved health, and clients can experience numerous benefits from Panchakarma treatment.

Benefits of Panchakarma therapy

Here are the benefits of Panchakarma:

Cleanses the digestive tract: Panchakarma cleanses the digestive tract by removing toxins and impurities from the body, which can help to improve digestion, reduce inflammation, and enhance overall gut health. This process can also help to prevent or alleviate gastrointestinal disorders such as bloating, constipation, and diarrhea.

Increases energy and vitality: By removing toxins and impurities from the body, Panchakarma can increase energy levels and vitality, leaving you feeling more rejuvenated and refreshed.

Balances the mind: Panchakarma helps to balance the mind and emotions by removing negative thought patterns and releasing emotional blockages. This can help to reduce stress, anxiety, and depression and promote a sense of peace and well-being.

Strengthens the immune system: Panchakarma stimulates the body's natural defenses by removing toxins and strengthening the immune system. This can help to prevent illness and disease and promote overall health and well-being.

Reduces stress and anxiety: Panchakarma helps to reduce stress and anxiety by promoting relaxation, reducing cortisol levels, and balancing the nervous system. This can also help improve sleep quality and promote overall well-being.

Improves digestion and assimilation: Panchakarma helps to improve digestion and assimilation by removing toxins and impurities from the body and strengthening the digestive system. This can help to alleviate digestive issues such as bloating, gas, and constipation.

Eliminates disease-causing free radicals: Panchakarma removes disease-causing free radicals from the body, which can help to prevent chronic diseases such as cancer and heart disease.

Strengthens the endocrine system: Panchakarma helps to balance and strengthen the endocrine system, which regulates hormones and plays a key role in overall health and well-being.

Creates clarity of mind: Panchakarma can help to create clarity of mind by removing mental and emotional blockages and promoting relaxation and calmness.

Releases negative emotions: Panchakarma can help to release negative emotions such as anger, resentment, and fear, leaving you feeling more balanced and at peace.

Reduces mental 'chatter': Panchakarma can help to reduce mental 'chatter' by promoting relaxation and calmness and improving focus and concentration.

Increases muscle strength and tone: Panchakarma can help increase muscle strength and tone by removing toxins and impurities from the body and promoting healthy tissue growth.

Strengthens and regenerates bone tissue: Panchakarma helps to strengthen and regenerate bone tissue by removing toxins and impurities from the body and promoting the growth of healthy bone tissue.

Balances the nervous system: Panchakarma therapy is known to positively affect the nervous system, promoting a sense of balance that helps reduce stress and anxiety. In addition, it can improve overall health and well-being, which may lead to increased happiness.

Decreases cholesterol: Panchakarma can help to decrease cholesterol levels by removing toxins and impurities from the body and promoting a healthy diet and lifestyle.

Unblocks arteries: Eliminating plaque and toxins from the body with the help of Panchakarma can improve circulation and lower the risk of heart disease by unblocking arteries.

Balances high and low blood pressure: Panchakarma can help to balance high and low blood pressure by removing toxins and impurities from the body and promoting a healthy diet and lifestyle.

The five treatments of Panchakarma

The five treatments that makeup Panchakarma are:

Vamana - Emesis Therapy: Involves induced vomiting with the help of medicinal herbs to remove the toxins from the upper respiratory and digestive tracts.

Virechana - Purgation Therapy: Involves induced bowel movements with the help of medicinal herbs to eliminate toxins from the liver and gastrointestinal tract.

Basti - Enema Therapy: Involves introducing medicinal liquids into the rectum to remove toxins from the colon and digestive tract.

Nasya - Nasal Administration: Involves the application of medicinal oils or powders to the nasal passages to remove toxins from the head and neck region.

Raktamokshana - Bloodletting Therapy: Involves the withdrawal of a small amount of blood from the body to remove toxins from the blood.

These comprehensive treatments involve several therapies performed over several days or weeks, depending on the individual's condition. Each treatment is designed to eliminate toxins from a specific body part, and the entire process is customized to suit the individual's needs.

Rasayana as a rejuvenation therapy

Rasayana is a powerful Ayurvedic therapy that aims to rejuvenate the mind, body, and spirit. The word "Rasayana" is derived from two Sanskrit words - "Rasa," meaning essence or vital fluid, and "Ayana," meaning path. Therefore, Rasayana therapy can be interpreted as the path to nourishing and revitalizing the body's essential fluid.

This therapy is based on the principles of Ayurveda and aims to promote health and longevity. According to Ayurveda, the human body comprises seven Dhatus or tissues, and the Rasa, or vital fluid, is the first. The Rasa is considered the most important as it nourishes and keeps the other six tissues balanced.

Rasayana therapy helps in replenishing the Rasa and other Dhatus, which helps in maintaining balance and preventing diseases. This therapy also helps in boosting the immune system and promotes the production of Ojas, which is considered the vital force of life in Ayurveda. Ojas is responsible for promoting strength, vitality, and immunity in the body.

After undergoing Panchakarma treatments, which are Ayurvedic detoxification therapies, rejuvenating herbal preparations, known as Rasayanas, are often prescribed to strengthen the immune system and increase vitality in the mind and body.

Types of Rasayana therapies

There are two main types of Rasayana therapies - Achara Rasayana and Aushadha Rasayana.

Achara Rasayana

Achara Rasayana is an important aspect of Ayurvedic rejuvenation therapy that involves making positive changes in one's lifestyle to promote health and longevity. Achara Rasayana primarily focuses on adopting healthy habits such as a balanced diet, regular exercise, proper sleep, stress management, and social engagement to maintain overall well-being.

One of the key aspects of Achara Rasayana is following a healthy diet rich in nutrients and antioxidants. Consuming fresh fruits, vegetables, whole grains, and lean proteins can help maintain optimal health and prevent the onset of chronic diseases. Avoiding processed foods, excessive sugar, and unhealthy fats can promote a healthy digestive system and boost immunity.

Regular exercise is another vital component of Achara Rasayana. Incorporating physical activity into one's daily routine can help improve cardiovascular health, boost metabolism, enhance mood, and increase strength and flexibility. Engaging in yoga, walking, swimming, or strength training can help maintain a healthy weight, prevent chronic diseases, and promote overall well-being.

Managing stress is also an important aspect of Achara Rasayana. Chronic stress can negatively impact the immune system, cardiovascular health, and mental well-being. Stress-reducing techniques such as meditation, deep breathing exercises, or engaging in creative activities can help manage stress and promote relaxation.

Lastly, social engagement and connection are essential aspects of Achara Rasayana. Staying connected with loved ones, engaging in meaningful activities, and volunteering in the community can help promote a sense of purpose, belonging, and fulfillment. This, in turn, can promote mental and emotional well-being and improve overall quality of life.

Aushadha Rasayana

Aushadha Rasayana is a type of rejuvenation therapy in Ayurveda that involves the use of specific herbal remedies and other natural substances to strengthen and revitalize the body. It is based on the principle that certain plants and natural substances possess rejuvenating properties that can help restore balance and vitality to the body's tissues, organs, and systems.

Herbal remedies used in Aushadha Rasayana are carefully selected based on their unique properties and ability to target specific health issues. For example, ashwagandha is known for its ability to help reduce stress and anxiety, while Amalaki is used to support digestion and promote healthy skin.

Other natural substances in Aushadha Rasayana include ghee, honey, and minerals. These substances are believed to have potent healing properties and are often used in Ayurvedic preparations to support overall health and wellness.

Aushadha Rasayana is typically recommended for individuals looking to improve their overall health and well-being, as well as those dealing with specific health concerns. It is often used in conjunction with other Ayurvedic therapies, such as Panchakarma and Achara Rasayana, to provide a comprehensive approach to health and wellness.

Benefits of Rasayana therapy

Rasayana therapies have numerous benefits for the body and mind, including:

Improved Immune Function: Rasayana therapies have immune-boosting properties that help to prevent disease and illness. These therapies help to improve the body's defense mechanisms and promote overall health and well-being.

Increased Energy and Vitality: Rasayana treatments help to restore energy and vitality to the body. These treatments improve the quality of life by promoting overall physical and mental well-being.

Reduced Stress: Stress is a major contributor to many health problems, such as heart disease, diabetes, and depression. Rasayana therapies help to reduce stress and promote relaxation, leading to improved overall health and well-being.

Better Digestion: Ayurvedic herbs and treatments can improve digestion, improving nutrient absorption and overall health. These herbs and treatments help to balance the digestive system and improve metabolism.

Enhanced Cognitive Function: Rasayana treatments can improve memory and cognitive function, helping to prevent age-related cognitive decline. These treatments promote mental clarity and alertness, improving overall cognitive health.

Anti-Aging Properties: Rasayana therapies can help to reduce the effects of aging on the body and mind, promoting a more youthful appearance and outlook on life. These therapies help to nourish and rejuvenate the body's cells, promoting overall health and vitality.

Improved Sleep: Ayurvedic herbs and treatments can improve sleep quality, improving overall health and well-being. These treatments help to promote relaxation and reduce stress, leading to improved sleep quality.

Better Skin Health: Many Ayurvedic herbs and treatments are known for their skin-healing properties, promoting healthy, glowing skin. These treatments help nourish and rejuvenate the skin, promoting overall health.

Increased Libido: Ayurvedic remedies can enhance sexual function and increase libido, improving the overall quality of life. These remedies help to balance the body's hormones and promote overall sexual health.

Rasayana herbs

Rasayana herbs are typically nourishing herbs rather than cleansing herbs. They can be difficult to digest if the body is suffering from an overload of toxins or if digestion is weak. These herbs are chosen for their specific properties that help restore the balance between body, mind, and spirit. Hence, the best time to take these powerful herbal formulas is after a course of Panchakarma treatments when the body has been cleansed and the digestion is functioning optimally. They can then be fully digested, assimilated, metabolized, and able to exert their full potential.

For optimal results with Rasayana formulas, it is best to use them consistently for a few months. Select formulas based on your Ayurvedic body type and the specific area of the body that requires attention. There are various traditional Rasayanas, each with unique benefits. Some nourish tissues, some rejuvenate, some enhance the immune system, some increase vitality and stamina, some balance the nervous system, and some strengthen the reproductive system.

Common Rasayana herbs

Here are some of the most common Rasayana herbs and their benefits:

Ashwagandha: This herb is known for its calming and rejuvenating effects. It is used to pacify and balance Vata, one of the three doshas (energies) in Ayurveda. Ashwagandha helps reduce stress, anxiety, and fatigue while promoting better sleep and overall well-being.

167

Amalaki: Also known as Indian gooseberry, Amalaki is a powerful antioxidant that helps improve digestion, boost the immune system, and enhance mental clarity. It is also known for its anti-aging properties and ability to balance pitta and Vata.

Brahmi: This herb is traditionally used for improving memory and cognitive function. It helps pacify pitta, which is responsible for heat and inflammation in the body. Brahmi is also known for its calming and relaxing effects on the mind and nervous system.

Turmeric: This bright yellow spice is known for its anti-inflammatory and antioxidant properties. It helps purify the blood, eliminate excess mucus, and soothe sore throats. Turmeric is also used to support healthy digestion and liver function.

Ginger, black pepper, and pippali: These herbs are often used together to improve digestion and pacify Kapha, which is responsible for congestion and sluggishness in the body. Ginger is also known for its anti-inflammatory properties, while black pepper and pippali help improve circulation and metabolism.

Aloe Vera: This succulent plant is known for its cooling and cleansing effects on the body. It helps cleanse the liver and blood while also balancing pitta. Aloe Vera is also used to support healthy skin and digestion.

Licorice: This sweet-tasting herb is known for balancing Vata, especially in the respiratory and digestive systems. Licorice helps soothe inflammation and promote healthy mucus production.

Peppermint: This refreshing herb balances Pitta and Kapha, making it an ideal herb for promoting overall balance and well-being. Peppermint helps support healthy digestion and reduce inflammation in the body.

Cinnamon, cayenne, ginger, and clove: These warming herbs are known to remove ama, a toxic substance that accumulates in the body due to poor digestion and metabolism. They also help improve circulation and metabolism while promoting overall balance and well-being.

Conclusion and Encouragement

As we come to the end of our transformative journey through "Ayurveda: The Science of Life," we have explored the profound wisdom and principles of Ayurveda, unlocking the path to healing and well-being. This book has offered us a deep understanding of Ayurveda's history, philosophy, and its relevance in our modern lives.

Throughout our exploration, we have recognized the fundamental elements of nature and their profound influence on our bodies and minds. By embracing the interconnectedness between these elements and us, we have gained a heightened awareness of the delicate balance that exists within us and the world around us.

Our journey has also illuminated the pivotal role of doshas in shaping our health and well-being. Through understanding our unique constitution, or prakriti, and the dynamic interplay between prakriti and vikriti, we have empowered ourselves to make conscious choices that restore harmony and prevent illnesses from taking hold.

The importance of digestion as the cornerstone of perfect health has been emphasized throughout the book. We have delved into the six tastes and their relationship to the elements, qualities, and doshas, enabling us to make mindful food choices that nourish and support our overall well-being. By nurturing a strong agni, the digestive fire, we unlock the innate healing potential of our bodies.

Furthermore, we have explored the cultivation of sattvic qualities, the detoxification of the mind, and the transformative power of mindfulness and meditation. By aligning ourselves with the rhythms of nature and honoring the influence of seasons and time of day on our well-being, we can prevent imbalances and foster holistic health.

The daily regimen of dinacharya and seasonal practices of ritucharya have been unveiled as invaluable tools for establishing a harmonious lifestyle. By embracing these regimens, we synchronize ourselves with the cycles of nature, optimizing our vitality and promoting well-being throughout the year.

In our final chapters, we have delved into the essence of doshas: ojas, tejas, and prana. We have explored their definitions, their impact on our overall well-being, and effective methods for increasing their presence within us. Additionally, we have highlighted the significance of reducing ama buildup, the toxic residue that can hinder our health and vitality.

As we conclude this transformative journey, I urge you, dear readers, to consider the profound benefits of yearly panchakarma therapy. Panchakarma serves as a powerful holistic detoxification and rejuvenation therapy, cleansing the body and revitalizing the mind. By undergoing the five treatments of panchakarma, you can release accumulated toxins, restore balance, and strengthen your immune system, effectively preventing the onset of various illnesses.

I invite you to embrace the wisdom of Ayurveda, integrating its principles into your life's tapestry. May this book be a guiding light on your journey to vibrant health, self-awareness, and inner harmony. Let Ayurveda be your trusted companion as you navigate the path to a life filled with wellness and vitality.

With heartfelt wishes for your continued well-being,

Alda Sainfort, MD, OMD, PgDA, MDiv.

Bibliography

Danny Cavanagh & Carol Willis. Everyday Ayurveda: A Practical Guide to Healthy Living. Ayurveda UK, 2004.

Kate O'Donnell. The Everyday Ayurveda Cookbook: A Seasonal Guide to Eating and Living Well. Shambhala Publications, 2015.

Susan Weis-Bohlen. Ayurveda Beginner's Guide: Essential Ayurvedic Principles and Practices to Balance & Heal Naturally. Althea Press, 2018.

Liebler N. C. & Moss S. Healing Depression the Mind-Body Way: Creating Happiness through Meditation, Yoga, and Ayurveda. John Wiley & Sons, Inc., 2009.

Johari H. Ayurvedic Healing Cuisine: 200 Vegetarian Recipes for Health, Balance, and Longevity. Healing Arts Press, 1994.

Lad V. The Complete Book of Ayurvedic Home Remedies. Three Rivers Press, 1998.

Rastogi S. Ayurvedic Science of Food and Nutrition. Springer, 2014.

Tirtha S. S. The Ãyurveda Encyclopedia: Natural Secrets to Healing, Prevention & Longevity. Ayurveda Holistic Center Press, 2005.

Lad V. D. Textbook of Ayurveda: Fundamental Principles of Ayurveda, Volume One. The Ayurvedic Press, 2002.

Mann T. Practical Ayurveda: Find Out Who You Are and What You Need to Bring Balance to Your Life. DK Publishing, 2018.

Resources

"An Invitation to Join Dr. Alda Sainfort on one of her Family Lineage Healing Retreats."

Advanced Healing Wellness Center
Visit our website: **www.ahwcenter.com** or
https://advancedhealingwellnesscenter.com/
Email us at **info@ahwcenter.com**
Call us 754-800-2391 or 954-900-1535

Book a Holistic Health Assessment & Evaluation

Book an Ayurvedic or Nutritional Assessment

Book a Panchakarma Therapy (Ayurvedic detox and rejuvenation)

Book a private or group spiritual healing / or family lineage healing session.

Join our upcoming Family Lineage Healing Retreat

Follow us

Facebook: **ahwcpines**

Instagram: **@ahwcpines**

https://tiktok.com/@advancedhealing

Subscribe to our YouTube channel:
https://www.youtube.com/@advancedhealingwellnesscen8701

Glossary

Abhyanga: is an Ayurvedic therapeutic bodywork involving massaging the body with warm oil to nourish and strengthen the body, calms the mind, and encourages regular sleep patterns.

Achara Rasayana: is a code of conduct that includes maintaining living standards based on honesty, trust, faith, love, and truth.

Adaptogen herbs: are a class of herbs that help the body adapt to stress and maintain balance or homeostasis. They regulate and establish balance in the hypothalamic, pituitary, and adrenal glands, which are involved in the stress response.

Agni: refers to the digestive and metabolic power of the body. It acts on receiving and converting nutrition into finer components.

Agni-enhancing: is considered a form of energy. The biological fire controls metabolism, digestion, and the immune system.

Akasha: It refers to Space and represents the essence of emptiness. It is the first and the most subtle of the five elements.

Alochak: is one of the five subtypes of Pitta; it is located in the eyes and responsible for vision.

Ama: is a term used for undigested food absorbed by the body but not digested.

Apana: This is one of the five subtypes of Vata, responsible for downward movement, like exhalation and excretion.

Arthava Veda: is a collection of prayers and ritual utterances written in early Sanskrit. It was added at a later stage to the existing Vedic material.

Ashtanga Hridayam: is one of the ancient core books of Ayurveda. It is known as the "Heart or Essence of all the eight Branches of Ayurveda." This text is still a foundation for Ayurvedic philosophy and protocol today, providing precise recommendations in all aspects of health.

Aushadha Rasayana: is a specialized treatment that helps maintain and promote health. The word "Rasayana" is composed of two words: "Rasa" and "Aayan." "Rasa" means "essence," and "Aayan" means "path". Rasayana therapy works as an immunomodulator for the prevention of various infectious diseases.

Avalamba: one of the subtypes of Kapha, located in the chest, protects the heart and supports the functions of the heart, lungs, and strong muscles.

Ayurveda: is a traditional Hindu system of medicine that emphasizes the importance of balance in bodily systems. The word "Ayurveda" is derived from Sanskrit; "Ayur" means "life" and "Veda" means knowledge or wisdom. It has been practiced for centuries and is based on the idea that the mind, body, and spirit are interconnected.

Basti: It refers to a type of treatment known as medicated enema therapy, derived from the Sanskrit word 'Basti', which means urinary bladder; this therapy involves the introduction of herbal decoctions and oils into the rectum to eliminate toxins and promote overall wellbeing.

Bhasrika: is a vital breath exercise in yoga and pranayama. It is sometimes treated as a kriya or 'cleansing action' along with kapalabhati to clear the airways in preparation for other pranayama techniques.

Bhrajak: one of the five subtypes of Pitta, located in the skin and responsible for imparting color, texture, and complexion to the skin.

Bhramari pranayama: a breathing technique that involves humming or buzzing sound during exhalation.

Bodhak: one of the subtypes of Kapha, located in the mouth and tongue, responsible for the sense of taste, which is essential for good digestion.

Buddhi: It is the four functions of the mind, and it refers to intellect, wisdom, and the power of the mind to understand, analyze, discriminate, and decide.

Charaka Samhita: is a Sanskrit text on Ayurveda. Along with the Sushruta Samhita, it is one of the two foundational texts of this field that have survived from ancient India.

Detoxification therapy refers to Panchakarma, a set of five treatments that help eliminate toxins from the body. The five Ayurvedic therapies that makeup Panchakarma are Vamana (Medicated Emesis), Virechana (Purgation), Nasya (Nasal Instillation), and Basti (Enema).

Dinacharya: refers to a daily routine meant to maintain physical health.

Dosha: is derived from the five elements and refers to three energies that define every person's makeup.

Drava: is a substance used to distill Ayurvedic medicines.

Greeshma: is a warm or hot and windy summer.

Guna: refers to the specific qualities or properties of all substances or things made of matter, including humans.

Guru: represents the heavy quality of a substance.

Hemanta: refers to winter, one of India's six seasons of the year.

Kapalabhati: is an energizing breathing practice that clears the lungs, the nasal passages, and the mind.

Kapha: Kapha types have strong frames and are naturally athletic as long they exercise regularly to manage their tendency to gain weight.

Kapha-pacifying: This diet consists of pungent, bitter, and astringent tastes while consuming lighter, warm, and easy-to-digest foods.

Kathina: is the characteristic of a drug referring to the hardness.

Khara: is the quality of roughness that protects against danger.

Kledak: located in the stomach, provides moisture to the stomach lining for good digestion.

Laghu: refers to the quality of lightness; its opposite is heaviness.

Macrocosm: refers to the entire universe, which contains may smaller systems known as microcosm

Mahagunas: Ayurveda identifies three mental states called Mahagunas: sattva, rajas, & tamas. They are at the core of skillful healing in Ayurveda.

Manda: refers to low-acting or dullness slow like in slow digestion or metabolism, known as manda agni.

Mantra: refers to powerful sound, chanting to produce healing through the increased vibration frequency in our body.

Microcosm: Ayurveda recognizes that every human being is a microcosm, a reflection of the macrocosm.

Mrudu: is the characteristic of a drug referring to soft.

Nadi shodhana: which refers to alternate nostril breathing" or channel cleaning breathing, is a pranayama breathing technique that aims to clear and purify the subtle channels of the mind-body organism while bringing balance to the whole body.

Ojas: refers to vigor, the vital energy that regulates our immunity, strength, and cheerfulness.

Pachak: one of the subtypes of Pitta; located in the stomach and intestines and responsible for digestion.

Panchakarma: is a set of five treatments that help eliminate toxins from the body. The five Ayurvedic therapies that make up Panchakarma are Vamana (Medicated Emesis), Virechana (Purgation), Nasya (Nasal Instillation), Basti (Enema).

Raktamokshana (Bloodletting): Panchakarma is an Ayurvedic set of five therapies that balance Doshas, strengthen Agni, detoxify ama, and rejuvenate the entire body.
Panchamahabhutas: refers to the five great elements that make up every element of this universe. These elements are Space, Air, Fire, Water, and Earth.

Paschat Karma (post-procedure care): refers to the actions taken after the primary Panchakarma treatments. It involves rejuvenation, formulations, recipes, dietary regimens, and lifestyle.

Pitta: Pitta types are dominated by the fire element, which makes them innately strong, intense, and irritable. They tend to be of medium build and endurance with powerful musculature.

Pitta-Kapha: it means that two doshas are predominant in the body constitution. Pitta embodies the transformative nature of Fire energy, while Kapha reflects the binding nature of Water energy.

Pitta-pacifying: means balancing Pitta with dietary regimen, daily and seasonal routines.

Pitta-Vata: it means that two doshas are predominant in the body constitution. Vata governs the flow of the breath, heart pulsation, muscle contractions, tissue movements, and communication throughout the mind. Pitta embodies the transformative nature of Fire energy.

Prabhav: This is the action that occurs when a substance has an unexpected and unexplained action, such as honey being sweet but heating rather than cooling.

Prajnaparadha: is one of the three crucial fundamental causes of diseases.

Prakriti: the innate, fixed body constitution established at conception.

Prana: life force, or vital energy that activates body and mind; it is known as qi in traditional Chinese medicine.

PranaVata: one of the five subtypes of Vata, it governs inhalation, perception through the senses, and controls the mind.

Pranayama: is the practice of breath regulation that is part of yoga. It involves breathing exercises that aim to control and manipulate the life force energy.

Pritvi: is the Sanskrit name for Earth.

Purusha: means Ayurveda and philosophical view. The soul represents pure consciousness or awareness. It is generally used to denote human beings.

Rajas: is one of the three gunas associated with activity, passion, change, and movement.

Raktamokshana means blood-letting therapy, an essential part of Panchakarma's clinical therapeutic use in managing some diseases or removing impure blood.

Rakta vaha srotas: are the channels transporting blood cells and specifically hemoglobin.

Ranjak: one of the five subtypes of Pitta, located in the liver and spleen.

Rasa: is the taste of food; the first experience of a food in the mouth. There are six rasa or six tastes: sweet, sour, salty, bitter, pungent, and astringent.

Rasayana: is Ayurvedic rejuvenation therapy that helps maintain and promote health.

Rejuvenation therapy: helps in the maintenance and promotion of health.

Ritucharya: is a lifestyle and diet designed to help cope with physical and mental impacts caused by seasonal changes.

Ruksha: means dry, one of the eight types of potency of medicinal herbs and one of the six therapeutic measures in Ayurveda.

Sad rasas: refers to the six tastes: sweet, sour, salty, pungent, bitter, and astringent.

Sadhaka Pitta: one of the subtypes of Pitta, located in the head/heart and responsible for emotions and thoughts.

Samana: one of the subtypes of Vata, governs peristaltic movement of the digestive system.

Sandra: is the quality of a drug referring to its thickness; its opposing quality, Drava, refers to its 'fluidity.'
Sanskrit: is the specific way to communicate the meaning of Ayurvedic terminologies.

Sara: refers to the essence of Dhatu with a smooth and excellent quality.

Sattva: is one of the three gunas; it represents beingness, harmony, balance, well-being, and intelligence.

Sharada: Sharada Shishira: late winter.

Shita refers to the cold quality, which increases Vata and Kapha and decreases Pitta.

Shleshak: one of the subtypes of Kapha, located in the bony joints, responsible for lubricating joints.

Shodana: is known as body purification therapy.

Snigdha: refers to one of the eight kinds of potency. It is oily, sticky, viscous or viscid, glutinous, soapy, slippery, smooth, glossy, greasy, treated or cured with oily substances adhesive.
Sthula: is one of the 20 gurvadi gunas caused by activated Prithvi (Earth). It indicates the physiological & pharmacological grossness & thickness.

Subdosha: Within each of the three doshas, five sub-doshas are responsible for managing specific actions, organs, or emotions.

Sukshma: means subtle or hidden. The presence of sukshma is felt but not seen.

Surya: means the Sun, the supreme source of energy and light.

Sushruta Samhita: is an ancient Sanskrit text on medicine and surgery and one of the most essential treatises to survive in the ancient world.

Tamas: is one of the gunas characterized by darkness, chaos, inertia, and materiality. Tamas can repress emotions, creating depression and anxiety and making our lives feel stuck. Tamasic foods include meat, oily, dense, stale, leftovers, etc.

Tapa: It refers to one of the five niyamas. It means taking time to be still to observe a deep state of meditation, which involves a high degree of self-discipline.

Tarpak: one of the subtypes of Kapha, located in the head, provides moisture for the nose, mouth, eyes, and brain.

Tejas: is the subtle form of fire of light in the body and mind. It is related to Pitta dosha, the constitution that governs intelligence, digestion, and the metabolic system.

Tivra: refers to very intense pleasure or fast.

Udana: one of the subtypes of Vata, governs speech, self-expression, enthusiasm, strength, and vitality.

Ushna: is the natural property of Pitta, which represents the fire inside and outside of the body.

Vamana: is an Ayurvedic therapy that eliminates excess Kapha (mucus) from the gastrointestinal and respiratory tract.

Varsha: is the season of monsoon that brings rain and relief from extreme summers.

Vasanta: is the Spring season, the time of renewal and rejuvenation.

Vata: tends to be thin and tall. They are mentally and physically active and enjoy creative endeavors, meeting new people, and traveling to new places.

Vata-Kapha: means two doshas are predominant in the body. Vata is the mobile nature of the Air, and Kapha reflects the binding nature of Water.

Vata-pacifying: Vata is cold and dry; a Vata pacifying diet involves a regular intake of foods that are warm, oily, moist, smooth, and nourishing to counteract the impact of Vata imbalance in the body.

Vata-Pitta-Kapha: The three body constitutions or doshas in Ayurveda are derived from the five elements: Space, Air, fire, Water, and Earth.

Veda: means knowledge, wisdom.

Vikriti: Vikriti refers to an individual's relative health or imbalance.

Vipak: describes the transformation of food after it is fully digested with the help of the digestive fire.

Virechana: is a procedure in the Panchakarma treatment. It involved the administration of purgative substances for the cleansing of Pitta through the lower pathways. It cleanses blood toxins, the sweat glands, kidneys, stomach, small intestine, colon, liver, spleen, and raktavaha srotas.

Virya: means the energy or potency of a drug or medicinal herbs.

Vyana: one of the subtypes of Vata, governs circulation and movement throughout the body.

About the Author

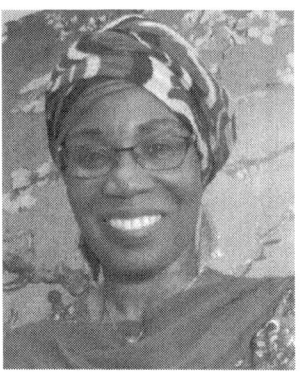

D r. Sainfort is a Board-Certified Holistic Care Specialist and founder of Advanced Healing Wellness Center in Pembroke Pines, Florida. The center has served the local and national communities for over a decade. She has dedicated over twenty-five years of her life to health and wellness, exploring and gaining a deep understanding of how to heal intergenerational or inherited pain, emotions, trauma, and patterns holistically.

After graduating from medical school with a degree in General Medicine, she began her career at the University of Miami Hospital & Jackson Health System in Investigative Clinical Trials in the departments of pediatrics, obstetrics, and gynecology, where she worked for almost five years. During her externship at the University of Miami Hospital in special immunology, surgery, neurology, obstetrics & gynecology, and pediatrics, she always wondered how medicines and therapies could heal patients conclusively.

In search of answers, Dr. Sainfort pursued her Post-Doctorate Studies in Ayurvedic medicine and Traditional Chinese Medicine/Acupuncture. She subsequently attended the University of Spiritual Healing and Sufism (USHS) in California and obtained a master's in divinity (M.Div.) with an emphasis on Spiritual Healing. Consequently, she has been continuously enrolled and studying Advanced Sufi Walking

(ASW) with Dr. Ibrahim Jaffe at the Institute of Spiritual Healing and other programs at the University of Sufism.

In 2004, She founded and funded Youth Operation Support, Inc., a non-profit organization to support troubled teenagers. She created after-school programs and activities to empower, inspire, and motivate them to stay in school and out of trouble.

As a healer, she has received insights that led her to research and deepen her knowledge by exploring, learning, and formulating different methods to address lineage-related emotional scars associated with inherited patterns, PTSD, or trauma. She continuously searched for truth and devoted many hours of research on ancestral relationships with the living.

Dr. Sainfort has been hosting family lineage healing retreats throughout the USA and other countries like India, promoting detoxification & rejuvenation therapy for many years. She has helped transform the health and lives of many, including adults, children, couples, and families with personal, intergenerational, and spiritual issues. Dr. Sainfort strongly believes and advocates a holistic approach to health and wellness.

Attending the University of Spiritual Healing and Sufism has opened a new door for her. The knowledge she acquired through the University has enhanced the multifold service experience to her clientele by encompassing the physical, emotional, and spiritual aspects to deliver complete healing. On many occasions, while working with clients, they would share their experience of seeing, connecting, or receiving messages from one or multiple ancestors: grandparents, great-grandparents, great-great-grandparents, or ancestors from many generations back. She has received divine guidance and insight on how to step in and carry the lineage healing legacy of her ancestors as a healer. She now incorporates a soul, spirit, and body approach to healing in her practice.

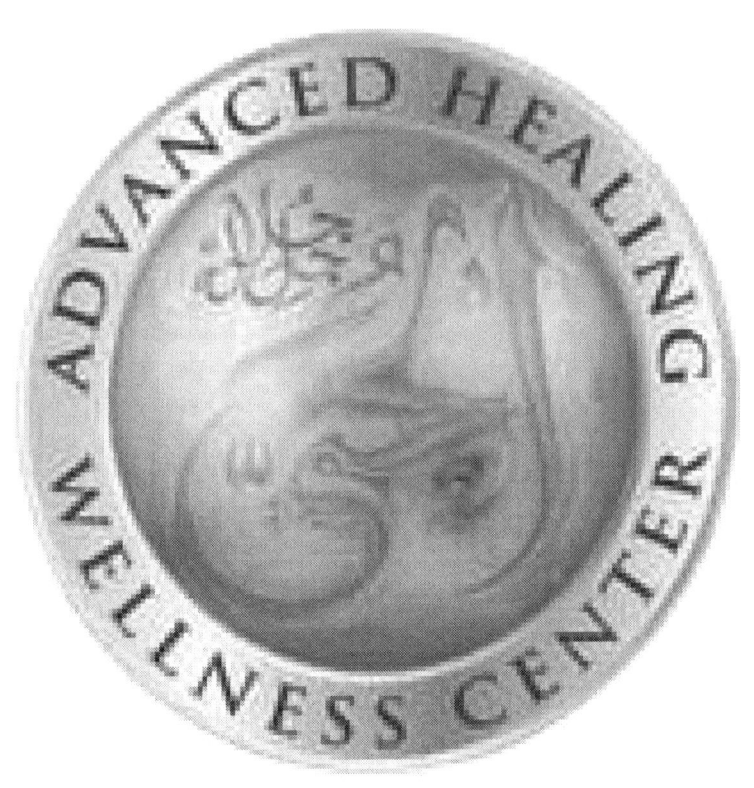

Made in the USA
Columbia, SC
19 October 2023

24232862R00111